Respiratory Insufficiency

Edited by Salim Surani,
Reena Shah and Syed Anjum Khan

Published in London, United Kingdom

Respiratory Insufficiency
http://dx.doi.org/10.5772/intechopen.105659
Edited by Salim Surani, Reena Shah and Syed Anjum Khan

Contributors
Eva Sánchez, Vijay Kant Pandey, Aaditya Anil Prabhudesai, Subhash Gupta, José Manuel Araiza Sánchez, Pedro Yasfir González-Noris, Juan Jose Espinoza-Espinosa, Marcos Alfonso Rosas, Alexey Gritsan, Mohammed Mohammednoor, Salim Surani, Muhammad K. Hayat Syed, Shehabaldin Alqalyoobi, Hillary Vaughan, Olalekan Bukunmi Ogunro, Oluwaseun Ruth Olasehinde

First published in London, United Kingdom, 2023 by IntechOpen
IntechOpen is the global imprint of INTECHOPEN LIMITED, registered in England and Wales, registration number: 11086078, 5 Princes Gate Court, London, SW7 2QJ, United Kingdom

British Library Cataloguing-in-Publication Data
A catalogue record for this book is available from the British Library

Additional hard and PDF copies can be obtained from orders@intechopen.com

Respiratory Insufficiency
Edited by Salim Surani, Reena Shah and Syed Anjum Khan
p. cm.
Print ISBN 978-1-83768-266-9
Online ISBN 978-1-83768-267-6
eBook (PDF) ISBN 978-1-83768-483-0

Meet the editors

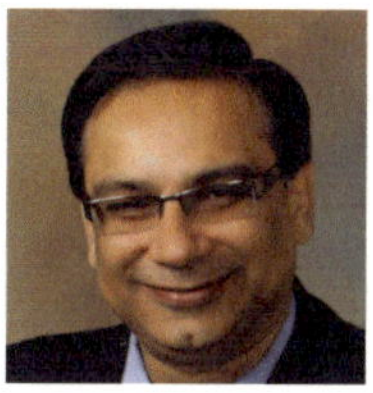

Dr. Salim Surani is an Adjunct Clinical Professor of Medicine, Department of Pulmonary, Critical Care & Sleep Medicine, Texas A&M University, USA, as well as a Clinical Professor of Pharmacology at Texas A&M University Kingsville. He is also a voluntary professor at the University of Houston, Texas, USA, and a research collaborator at Mayo Clinic, Minnesota, USA. He serves as the director of the Pulmonary Fellowship Program at Bay Area Medical Center, Corpus Christi, Texas, USA. He completed a fellowship in pulmonary medicine at Baylor College of Medicine, Houston, Texas, USA. Dr. Surani received a master's degree in Public Health and Epidemiology from Yale University and a master's degree in Health Management from the University of Texas, Dallas, USA. Dr. Surani also has served as a board trustee and secretary for the CHEST Foundation and chair of the practice operations network of the American College of Chest Physicians (ACCP). He is on the award committees for ACCP and the American Academy of Sleep Medicine (AASM). He is editor-in-chief, editorial board member, and reviewer for several peer-reviewed journals. He has served on the steering committee for the executive committee of networks of ACCP. Dr. Surani has authored more than 300 articles in peer-reviewed journals and has written several books and book chapters. He has been involved in teaching residents for more than two decades and has received numerous Faculty of the Year awards. He has established himself as a Master Clinician who has trained significant numbers of practicing primary care, internal medicine, and emergency physicians in the Coastal Bend region. Dr. Surani has established several ICU-intensivist models in the region and has served in every possible leadership role in the hospital system. He has also helped start an emergency medicine residency program. He has served as a speaker at several regional, national, and international scientific conferences. His areas of expertise include critical care, sleep medicine, ICU infections, and practice operations. He has also served on committees for several national organizations and has received several community and teaching awards, including the Health Care Hero award and humanitarian awards from the American College of Physicians, ACCP, and Texas Medical Association. Dr. Surani is highly regarded among his peers and is very well respected as a mentor, clinician, and humanitarian.

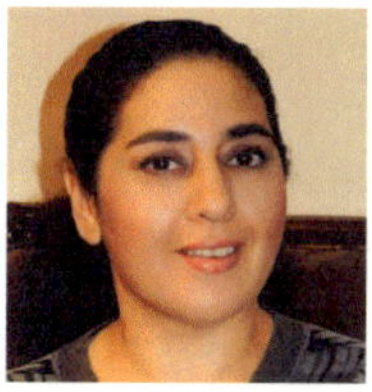

Dr. Syed Anjum Khan has been involved in patient care, education, and curriculum development for critical care education for more than two decades. She has served as the regional chair of the critical care division of the Southwest Minnesota Mayo Clinic Health System since 2007. She is also a member of the organization's specialty critical care council committee. In addition, she is a member of the Mayo Clinic Enterprise critical care specialty council and practice committee. Dr. Khan played an instrumental role in taking care of critically ill covid patients during the COVID-19 pandemic and was the site investigator for the Discovery virus trial, which was a collaboration between the Society of Critical Care Medicine and the Mayo Clinic. Dr. Khan is an exceptional educator, researcher, mentor, and critical care physician.

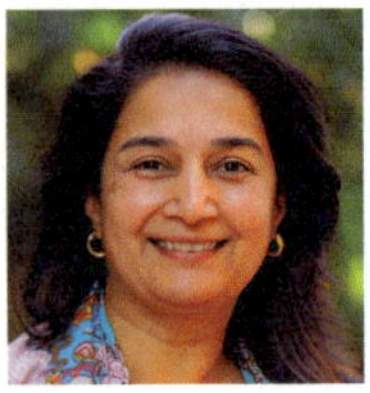

Prof. Reena Shah is a consultant physician, section head of infectious diseases, and the fellowship director for the infectious disease fellowship program at Aga Khan University Hospital in Nairobi, Kenya. She has recently been appointed head of the Department of Medicine at the same hospital. She received her MBBS from the University of Southampton, UK in 1996 and her MRCP from the Royal College of Physicians London in 2000. She obtained a diploma in Infectious Diseases from the University of London, UK in 2008 as well as a diploma in Tropical Medicine and Infectious Diseases from the London School of Tropical Medicine and Hygiene in 2009. She also holds a master's degree in Infectious Diseases from the University of London. She obtained a fellowship from the Royal College of Physicians Edinburgh (FRCPE) in 2014 and a fellowship from the Royal College of Physicians London (FRCP) London in 2018. Dr. Shah is currently leading Aga Khan University Hospital in COVID-19 response as the head of infectious diseases and a frontline worker. She has also been involved in the development of the national case management guidelines in Kenya. With her new appointment, she oversees all sections of internal medicine, including cardiology, pulmonology, gastroenterology, neurology, intensive care, and others.

Contents

Preface

Adequate oxygenation and carbon dioxide removal are integral parts of respiratory system homeostasis. In respiratory failure, one or both of these vital functions are compromised. Respiratory failure can be due to pump failure manifested by hypercapnia and lung failure manifested by gas exchange failure and hypoxemia. Four pathophysiological mechanisms can lead to respiratory failure: ventilation-perfusion mismatch, shunt, diffusion impairment, and alveolar hypoventilation [1, 2]. Incidence of respiratory failure is 137.1/100,000, with mortality as high as 29%–42%. In the United States in 2017, there were approximately 1,146,195 patients discharged from the hospital with the diagnosis of respiratory failure, with an average length and hospital charge of 10.5 days and a cost per admission of $158,493 [3, 4]. While the incidence of cardiovascular disease is decreasing, the incidence and prevalence of respiratory illness, including obstructive lung disease, is on the rise. Globally, 545 million people live with respiratory illness, representing 7.4% of the world's population. Chronic obstructive pulmonary disease is the third leading cause of death globally, with 3.2 million deaths in 2019. In addition, there were 495,000 deaths due to asthma [5]. Respiratory illness accounts for 20% of all mortality. In addition, the COVID-19 pandemic created global havoc with the SARS-CoV2 virus causing respiratory failure and associated high mortality. COVID patients who required mechanical ventilation had an increased risk of death [6, 7].

This book provides a comprehensive overview of respiratory insufficiency. In the first section, Chapter 1 discusses the pathophysiology of respiratory failure. It addresses the anatomy and physiology of the respiratory system and examines lung volume, capacities, and changes during obstructive and restrictive lung disease. In addition, it discusses the pathophysiology of hypoxemia and hypercapnia and the physiological response to the pathologies.

Section 2 discusses respiratory failure in obstructive lung disease. Chapter 2 discusses acute respiratory failure exacerbating bronchial asthma. The chapter reviews the pathogenesis of asthma, early and late response to antigens, airway remodeling phenomenon, and other factors such as microbiome and microbiota. It also discusses dynamic hyperinflation and its predisposing factors. Chapter 3 on respiratory support in obstructive syndrome discusses the biomechanics and gas exchange in acute respiratory failure, respiratory support, and its algorithm. It also discusses the challenges for patients with mechanical ventilation.

Section 3 addresses issues in patients with respiratory failure due to COVID-19. As mentioned, patients with respiratory failure due to COVID-19 have high mortality. Chapter 4 discusses the clinical manifestation and management of respiratory failure in COVID patients as compared to that in non-COVID-19 patients.

Section 4 addresses respiratory failure in specialized conditions, including in patients with liver disease, and the management of mechanical ventilation in burn patients, which carries a high mortality. Chapter 5 discusses porto-pulmonary hypertension and hepatopulmonary syndrome. It discusses the clinical features, diagnosis, and management of these conditions as well as the role of liver transplant in patients with hepatopulmonary syndrome. Chapter 6 discusses airway management in burn patients, including those with carbon monoxide and cyanide toxicity and inhalation injury. It also reviews the diagnosis and mechanical ventilation management among burn patients.

The book concludes with Section 5 on the role of veno-venous extracorporeal membrane oxygenation (VV-ECMO) in respiratory failure. Chapter 7 discusses the physiology of VV-ECMO as well as its management and complications. It also discusses the role of VV-ECMO in patients with acute respiratory distress syndrome (ARDS) due to COVID-19.

This book provides an understanding of the basic physiology and management of patients with respiratory insufficiency. It discusses specialized populations with respiratory failure and the role of VV-ECMO. We hope that readers will find this book useful and informative.

Salim Surani, MD, MPH, MSHM, FACP, FCCP, FAASM, FCCM
Clinical Professor,
Texas A&M University,
College Station,
Texas, USA

Visiting Professor,
Aga Khan University,
Nairobi, Kenya

Syed Anjum Khan, MD
Regional Chair of Critical Care Medicine,
Southwest Minnesota Mayo Clinic Health System,
Minnesota, USA

Reena Shah, MD, MRCP (lon), DTM&H, MScID (Lon), FRCP(Edin), FRCP(Lon)
Associate Professor and Chief of Medicine,
Aga Khan University,
Nairobi, Kenya

References

[1] Roussos C, Koutsoukou A. Respiratory failure. The European respiratory journal Supplement. 2003;**47**:3s-14s

[2] Gandhi KD, Sharma M, Taweesedt PT, Surani S. Role of proning and positive end-expiratory pressure in COVID-19. World J Crit Care Med. 2021;**10**(5):183-93

[3] Kempker JA, Abril MK, Chen Y, Kramer MR, Waller LA, Martin GS. The Epidemiology of Respiratory Failure in the United States 2002-2017: A Serial Cross-Sectional Study. Crit Care Explor. 2020;**2**(6):e0128

[4] Viegi G, Maio S, Fasola S, Baldacci S. Global Burden of Chronic Respiratory Diseases. J Aerosol Med Pulm Drug Deliv. 2020;**33**(4):171-7

[5] Organization WH. Chronic Obstructive Lung Disease: World Health Organization; 2023 [Available from: https://www.who.int/news-room/fact-sheets/detail/chronic-obstructive-pulmonary-disease-(copd)

[6] Barria-Sandoval C, Ferreira G, Mendez A, Toffoletto MC. Impact of COVID-19 on deaths from respiratory diseases: Panel data evidence from Chile. Infect Ecol Epidemiol. 2022;**12**(1):2023939

[7] Asghar MS, Yasmin F, Haris A, Nadeem A, Taweesedt PT, Surani S. Comparison of first and second waves of COVID-19 through severity markers in ICU patients of a developing country. J Community Hosp Intern Med Perspect. 2021;**11**(5):576-84

Section 1

Pathophysiology of Respiratory Failure

Chapter 1

Pathophysiology of Respiratory Insufficiency

Mohammed Mohammednoor

Abstract

This chapter will discuss the pathophysiology of the two types of respiratory failure type 1 and type 2, also known as hypoxic type and hypercapnic type respectively, which will help in understanding how respiratory diseases emerge. The next few pages will go through anatomy, physiology, and mechanisms of developing hypoxia and hypercapnia. This will be the fundamental of respiratory diseases. Diseases that can cause any type of respiratory failure will be mentioned without going into detail as it has a separate chapter. Hypoxia can be caused by V/Q mismatch, right-to-left shunt, and diffusion restriction. Hypoventilation can result in both hypoxic and/or hypercapnic types.

Keywords: respiratory failure, respiratory insufficiency, pathophysiology, hypoxemia, hypercapnia

1. Introduction

This chapter will shed light on the pathophysiology of respiratory failure or the new term respiratory insufficiency to understand how respiratory diseases emerge, their complications, and management. This chapter will include the anatomy and physiology of the lungs, the pathophysiology of respiratory insufficiency, and the interpretation of ABG.

2. Anatomy of the respiratory system

2.1 General

The respiratory tract can be categorized into upper and lower or conduction and gas exchange parts (**Figure 1**).

1. Upper vs. Lower

   The upper respiratory tract includes the nasal cavity, paranasal sinuses, pharynx, and larynx above the vocal cord.

   The lower respiratory tract includes the larynx below vocal cords, trachea, bronchi, and lungs (bronchioles and alveoli) [1].

2. Conduction vs. Ventilation (Gas exchange)

Conduction includes all parts from the nose to the terminal bronchioles.

Gas exchange includes respiratory bronchioles and alveoli.

2.2 Blood supply

Lungs receive arterial blood supply from both bronchial arteries branches of the thoracic aorta (oxygenated blood) and pulmonary artery originating from the right

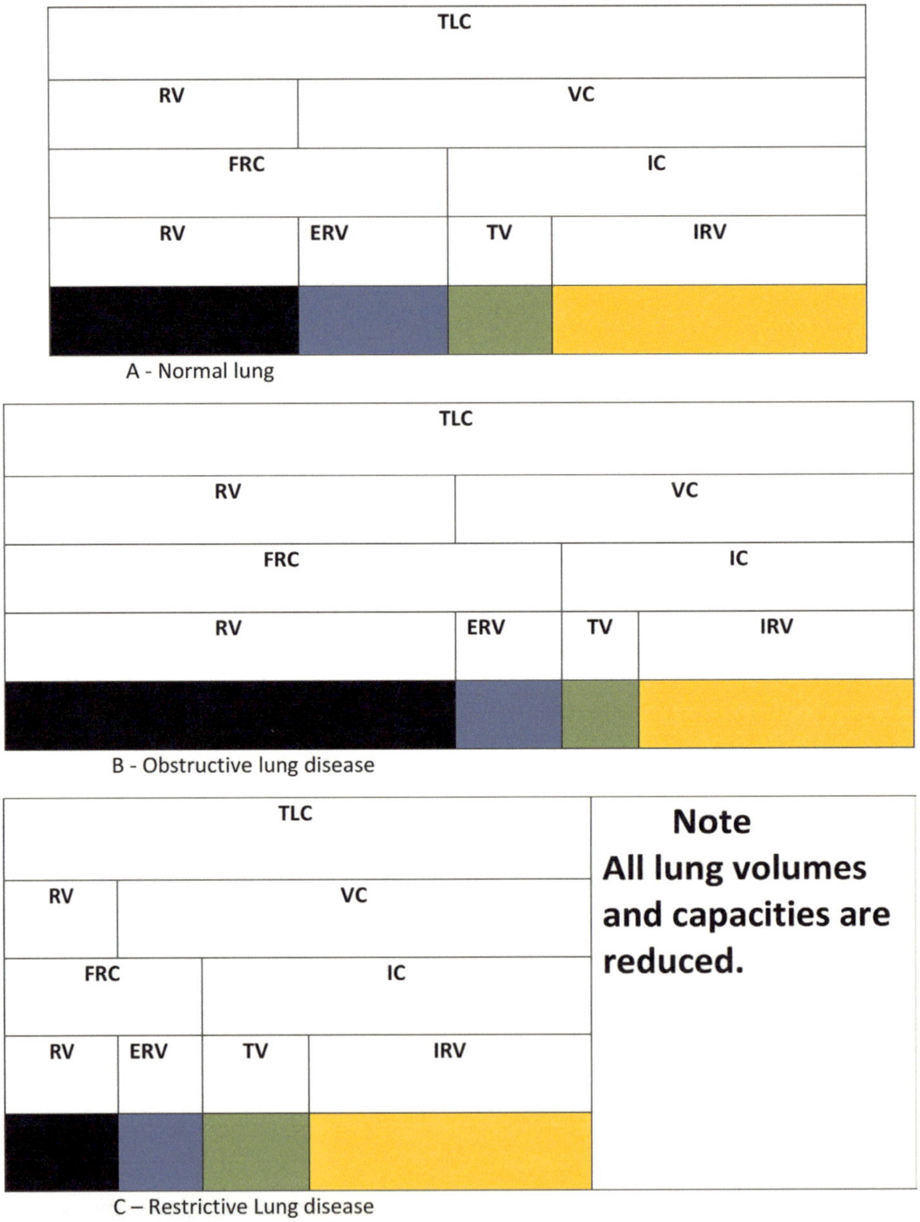

Figure 1.
This figure illustrates the difference between a; Normal lung function, B: Obstructive lung diseases, C: Restrictive lung diseases. Note the change of width of different lung function parameters.

ventricle of the heart (deoxygenated blood for gas exchange). Venous drainage via bronchial veins (deoxygenated blood) which drain into the azygos vein (right) and left superior costal vein or hemiazygos vein (left) and pulmonary veins (oxygenated blood) which drain into the left atrium [1].

2.3 Nerve supply

Respiratory system is supplied primarily by sympathetic and parasympathetic fibers originated from pulmonary plexuses which lie anterior and posterior to the lungs roots, it provide supply to the smooth muscles of the bronchial tree, the vessels and the mucus membranes [1].

2.4 Lymphatic drainage

Bronchopulmonary lymph nodes at the bifurcation of the large bronchi drain lungs and visceral pleural lymphatic that then passes to hilar tracheobronchial nodes, which drain into the broncho mediastinal trunk on each side [1].

3. Physiology of the respiratory system

Gas exchange between the alveolus and the blood capillary depends on the passive diffusion of PO_2 in the alveolus (around 100 mmHg), and the blood entering the capillary (around 40 mm). This difference results in the diffusion of O_2 from the alveolus to the capillaries. The barrier to this process includes a cytoplasmic extension of type 1 cells, the basement membrane, and the capillary endothelial layer. CO_2 diffuses more readily than O_2 because of its high plasma solubility [2].

Another important part of lung physiology is compliance which simply means the opposite of stiffness. During inspiration, contraction of the diaphragm creates negative pressure around the lungs allowing the lungs to expand in addition to the positive pressure exerted on the lungs from the airways. Thus, the difference between the positive pressure (from airways) exerted on alveoli, and negative pressure in the pleural space is called transpulmonary pressure. So, the compliance relationship (pressure-volume relationship) between transpulmonary pressure and the volume inside the lungs can be represented by a curve that flattens at high distending pressure when the lungs reach their upper limit of expansion. That means the elastic tissue of the lungs at this point cannot be stretched further, and no additional volume of air can be added [2].

So, diseases affecting the alveoli may disrupt compliance making the lung either stiffer (more resistant to expansion) or less stiff (easily expandable). For stiff lungs (less compliance), the curve is shifted to the right, so lower volume is achieved for any transpulmonary pressure. So, patients with more compliant lungs shift the curve to the left, and higher volume can be achieved with low pressure [2]. as shown in **Figure 1**, changes in lung volumes in obstructive vs. restrictive vs. normal lung [2].

Airway resistance is inversely proportional to lung volumes which means during inspiration, airway resistance decreases, especially in small bronchioles, to enhance expansion. Conversely, airway resistance increases during forceful expiration due to flow-limiting segments [2].

Given the compliance, the lung can have different volumes and capacities as shown in **Table 1** and **Figure 1**.

Volume/capacity	Definition	Normal values
Tidal volume (TV)	amount of air passing into and out of the lungs during breathing.	300–500 ml (6–8 ml/kg)
Inspiratory reserve volume (IRV)	the extra volume of air that can be inhaled into the lungs during maximal inspiration, i.e., over and above normal TV	1900–3300 ml
Expiratory reserve volume (ERV)	the volume of air that can be expelled from the lungs during maximal expiration	700–1200 ml
Residual volume (RV)	the volume of air remaining in the lungs after forced expiration.	approximately 1200 ml (20–25 ml/kg)
Inspiratory capacity (IC)	amount of air that can be inspired with maximum effort IC = TV + IRV	2200–3800 ml
Vital capacity (VC)	the maximum amount of air a person can expel from the lungs after a maximum inhalation. VC = IC + ERV	approximately 4800 ml
Functional Residual Capacity (FRC)	Amount of the air remaining in the lung after normal expiration FRC = RV + ERV	1800–2200 ml
Total lung capacity (TLC)	The maximum amount of air the lungs can accommodate TLC = VC + RV	4–6 L

Table 1.
Definition of lung volumes and normal ranges.

In normal adults, only 70% of tidal volume (350 ml) is available to exchange as 30% remains in what is called anatomical dead space (150 ml) (which extends from nose to terminal bronchioles).

4. Pathophysiology of hypoxemia and hypercapnia

4.1 Pathophysiology of hypoxemia

Hypoxemia can be defined as $PaO_2 < 10.6$ kPa. Also known as lung failure.
Alveolar – Arterial Oxygen Gradient:
It's the difference between alveolar oxygen level (A) and arterial oxygen level (a).
A-a: $PAO_2 - PaO_2$, it is simply reflecting the integrity of the alveolocapillary membrane and the effectiveness of gas exchange:

$PAO_2 = FiO_2 \times (Pb - PH_2O) - (PACO_2/R)$
PAO_2 = mean alveolar oxygen pressure.
FiO_2 = fractional concentration of inspired Oxygen. Which is 021 in room air.
Pb = barometric pressure (760 mmHg at sea level).
PH_2O = water vapor pressure (47 mmHg at 37 C).
$PACO_2$ = alveolar Pressure of CO_2, which is almost equal to $PaCO_2$.
R = respiratory quotient and is approximately 0.8 at steady state on the standard diet.
From this, normal $PAO_2 = 0.21 \times (760\text{–}47) - (40/0.8) = 100$ mmHg.

Table 2.
PAO_2 is not measured unlike PaO_2, but it is calculated using the following equation.

Hypoxemia with a normal A-a gradient indicates hypoventilation, whereas a High A-a gradient indicates V/Q mismatch, diffusion restriction, and shunt. See **Table 2**, how to calculate alveolar oxygen pressure.

A-a difference is <10 mmHg in young people, but it increases with age due to an increase in V/Q mismatch. It is estimated that after 70 years of age, PaO_2 drops by 0.43 mmHg every year. A high gradient indicates high FiO_2, which increases both alveolar and arterial oxygenation, but arterial O_2 pressure does not increase in the same proportion to the alveolar O_2 pressure due to mixing with deoxygenated blood from Bronchial veins and mediastinal veins.

Also referred to as Type 1 respiratory failure, it can be divided into four categories

1. V/Q mismatch.

   It is the commonest mechanism for hypoxemia, normal V/Q level is 0.8. it varies across the lung where apexes are well-ventilated and poorly perfused, which means a higher V/Q ratio. And bases are well perfused than ventilated, giving low V/Q. This explains why the apical region has higher O_2, and low CO_2 and bases have low O_2 and high CO_2 content [3].

   Parts of the lungs where there is a low Ventilation-perfusion ratio return more deoxygenated blood to the systemic circulation. i.e., fluid-filled alveoli or airway disease impairs the ventilation of alveoli. e.g., pneumonia, or the broad term ARDS (acute respiratory distress syndrome), where there is an increase in permeability of pulmonary capillaries leading to increase extravasation of fluids to the surrounding tissue and alveoli [4].

   The normal physiological response of pulmonary vasculature to poorly-ventilated regions is constriction and diversion of blood to well-ventilated areas (this creates shunting), but that can fail to compensate in extreme situations and lead to hypoxia. This physiological response is called Hypoxic pulmonary vasoconstriction (HPV).

   HPV is a protective mechanism to maintain a normal ventilation/perfusion ratio. But it has a negative consequence in chronic cases as it can lead to chronic pulmonary hypertension. As shown in **Table 3**, the mechanism of development of HPV.

   Characteristics of high V/Q mismatch [4]:

   - Hypoxemia is easily treated by increasing FiO_2. Hence supplemental oxygen therapy.
   - Widened A-a Gradient can indicate a high V/Q mismatch.
   - Examples of common diseases that can result in hypoxemia due to V/Q mismatch are asthma, COPD, bronchiectasis, cystic fibrosis, interstitial lung disease (ILD), pneumonia, and pulmonary hypertension. Note most of these diseases can progress to type 2 respiratory failure.

2. Right-to-left shunt [4].

   Right-to-left shunt means blood from the right side of the heart (deoxygenated) mixes with blood in the left side circulations (oxygenated). Normally there is a

• The inhibition of the oxygen-sensitive potassium channel initiates the process of HPV. • Hypoxia inhibits the voltage-gated K+ channels present in the pulmonary artery leading to the accumulation of intracellular K+ and depolarization of the cells. • Depolarization opens the voltage-gated L-Type Ca2+ channels resulting in Ca2+ influx and subsequently results in vasoconstriction.

Table 3.
Mechanism of HPV.

2% fraction due to anastomosis between bronchial veins carrying deoxygenated blood and pulmonary veins carrying oxygenated blood.

Shunt is considered an extreme form of V/Q mismatch where there is no ventilation. It has a poor response to oxygen therapy, so the failure to increase PaO_2 is due to the failure of delivering O_2 (PAO_2) to unventilated parts of the lung. It can progress to hypercapnia when the shunt fraction is>50%. Lack of hypercapnia is due to stimulation of the respiratory center by chemoreceptors as a result of an increase in $PaCO_2$.

Characteristics of pulmonary shunt:

- P (A-a) O_2 is elevated
- Poor response to oxygen therapy
- PCO_2 is normal until the late stages
- Examples of common diseases associated with a shunt are pneumonia, ARDS, alveolar collapse, and pulmonary arteriovenous communications.

3. Diffusion restriction

It means diffusion of O_2 across the alveolocapillary membrane is reduced due to a decrease in alveolar surface area as a result of inflammation, fibrosis, low alveolar oxygen, and short capillary transit time.

As both O_2 and CO_2 diffuse through the membrane during gas exchange, low permeability should result in both hypoxemia and hypercapnia, but that is not the case since CO_2 is 20 times more soluble than O_2, hence less likely affected by diffusion restriction [3].

Normal gas exchange time is 0.25 sec, whereas capillary transit time is 0.75 sec. So, diffusion restriction can result in the development or worsening of hypoxemia during exercise. This can be explained as a shortening of capillary transit time during exercise due to the rise of CO. Additionally, venous O_2 level drops due to increased oxygen consumption by tissues. In a normal person, that usually does not happen as compensatory mechanisms come into action, such as recruitment of the capillaries, distention of capillaries, and increase in PAO_2. Thus, patients with pulmonary fibrosis are unable to recruit more capillaries which results in exercise-induced hypoxemia [3].

Characteristics of diffusion restriction:

- Good response to oxygen therapy
- A-a gradient is elevated
- $PaCO_2$ is normal
- Examples of common causes of hypoxemia due to diffusion limitations are emphysema and ILD.

4. Hypoventilation [4]

Ventilation contributes to oxygenation and CO_2 washout; thus, the hallmark of hypoventilation is a rise in $PaCO_2$ and the development of hypercapnia, i.e., type 2 respiratory failure. But initially, hypoventilation results in low PAO_2 and eventually hypoxemia (low PaO_2), i.e., type 1 respiratory failure. As mentioned earlier, hypoventilation is associated with normal A-a gradient but not exclusively, as prolonged hypoventilation can cause atelectasis which leads to the widening of the A-a gradient [4].

Normal pulse oximetry indicates adequate ventilation (normal $PaCO_2$) in the patient's breathing room air, but it is difficult to interpret in a patient on supplemental oxygen, as hypoventilation may persist. In other words, hypoventilation-induced hypoxemia is responsive to supplemental oxygen but does not mean correction of $PaCO_2$ as well.

COPD, asthma, and ILD patients initially develop type 1 respiratory insufficiency, but after a period, it can progress to type 2 respiratory failure due to the retention of $PaCO_2$.

Alveolar gas equation [4]:

$$PaCO2 = K \frac{V'CO2}{VT\,X\,RR\,\left(1 - \frac{VD}{VT}\right)} \quad (1)$$

$PaCO_2$ = arterial partial pressure of CO_2.
$V'CO_2$ = CO_2 production in the body.
K = Factor (0.863) is constant.
V_T = tidal volume.
RR = respiratory rate.
VD = Dead space Ventilation.
Note:

- VT X RR = minute ventilation (V'E).
- Alveolar Ventilation (V'A) = V'E − V'D.

Thus, the reasons for the increase in $PaCO_2$ could be due to the increased production of CO_2 by the body ($V'CO_2$). Without a compensatory rise in alveolar ventilation (V'A), rise in dead space ventilation VD, and drop in RR and/or VT.

A-a oxygen gradient can help differentiate whether the high $PaCO_2$ is due to the reduction in VT or an increase in VD. The gradient will be normal on VT reduction and high in increased VD. If compensatory functions are normal, increased body production of CO_2 will not increase $PaCO_2$.

Conditions that may raise body production of CO_2 are burns, sepsis, exercise, hyperthermia, intake of carbohydrate-rich diet, tetanus, seizures, and tremor.

Conditions that may give rise to VD/VT ratio are PE, COPD, ARDS, and Bronchiectasis.

Mechanism of Hypoventilation:

Hypoventilation arises from respiratory dysfunction at various levels; hence it can be divided into central and peripheral causes:

1. Central: - impaired central drive

    i. Brain stem: hemorrhage or infarction

    ii. Drugs overdose: opioids, benzodiazepines, alcohol

    iii. Primary alveolar hypoventilation

    iv. Spinal cord level: amyotrophic lateral sclerosis, cervical spinal cord injury.

2. Peripheral:

    i. Nerve supplying respiratory muscles: Guillain–Barre syndrome

    ii. Neuromuscular junction: Myasthenia gravis, Lambert–Eaton syndrome

    iii. Respiratory muscles: Myopathy

    iv. Defects in chest wall: Kyphoscoliosis, thoracoplasty, fibrothorax.

Characteristics of hypoventilation:

- Hypoxemia has a good response to supplemental oxygen.
- A-a gradient is usually normal
- $PaCO_2$ will eventually rise if hypoventilation persists.

4.1.1 Essential measurements for hypoxemia

Arterial oxygen partial pressure: PaO_2 indicates dissolved oxygen, not hemoglobin-bound oxygen. It is measured by an arterial gas analyzer.

In mixed venous blood, PaO_2 is 40 mmHg, 75% saturation. On the other hand, in arterial blood, it is 97% saturation. It never gets to 100% saturation as the presence of anatomical dead space.

Arterial oxygen content (CaO_2) is the summation of hemoglobin-bound oxygen and the dissolved oxygen in the arterial blood. The following equation calculates it

$$CaO_2 = (Hgb \times 1.34 \times SaO_2) + (0.0031 \times PaO_2). \quad (2)$$

From the above equation, it can be noted that dissolved PaO_2 has minimal contribution to the arterial oxygen content, which explains normal PaO_2 in anemia.

Arterial oxygen saturation (SaO_2): means the percentage of hemoglobin saturated with oxygen. It can be measured by both pulse oximetry and gas analyzer.

PaO_2/FiO_2 ratio: it is the ratio of partial pressure of oxygen in arterial blood to the fraction of inspired oxygen. The normal ratio is between 300 and 500 mmHg. It plays a major role in prognostication in ARDS patients. ARDS is categorized into mild (PaO_2/FiO_2 ratio 200–300 mmHg, moderate 100–200 mmHg, and severe PaO_2/FiO_2 < 100 mmHg). As mentioned earlier, it can be used to estimate shunt fraction. A PaO_2/FiO_2 ratio of <200 indicates a shunt fraction is more than 20%.

4.2 Pathophysiology of hypercapnia

On the other hand, hypercapnia, defined as an increase in $PaCO_2 > 6$ kPa, also can be referred to as pump failure. And the mechanism of development of hypercapnia can be divided into four categories:

1. Decreased minute ventilation (i.e., hypoventilation) which can be due to central or peripheral causes (see above).

2. Increased dead space

3. Increase CO_2 production

4. Multifactorial.

Decreased minute ventilation: It has been discussed earlier in the pathophysiology of hypoxemia [3].

4.2.1 Increased dead space

Dead space is defined as the area of the lung that is unable to provide gas exchange, whether anatomically or physiologically incapable.

There are two types of dead space anatomical (from nose to bronchi), and physiologic dead space which is equal to the summation of anatomical dead space and alveolar dead space (volume of air in the alveolar that does not participate in gas exchange).

Anatomical dead space represents 30% of tidal volume which is roughly equal to 150 ml.

Tachypnea which could contribute to washing out CO_2 from blood can also participate in hypercapnia by increasing dead space to tidal volume ratio VD/Vt. High alveolar ventilation (VA) and associated with V/Q mismatch are considered the main reasons for hypercapnia in COPD patients [3].

4.2.2 Increased CO_2 production

As we know, CO_2 is a by-product of oxidative metabolism. Thus, any increase in metabolic status can lead to an increase in CO_2, such as fever/sepsis, exercise, total parenteral nutrition, and thyrotoxicosis. In the normal respiratory system, this rise in CO_2 production is well compensated by the rise in minute ventilation, but that may become pathological if there is a failure of the compensatory mechanism.

Normal young adult production of CO_2 ($V'CO_2$) is around 200 $mL.min^{-1}$ or 110 ml in males and 96 ml in females. It increases by 14% for each degree Celsius rise in temperature [5].

5. Physiological response to hypoxia

5.1 Physiological response to hypoxia

The body's response to low levels of oxygen in the blood can be divided into two [5]:

1. Systemic response:

   - Several chemosensory systems act in sync during reduced availability of O_2 by modulating ventilation, perfusion, and blood circulation to optimize oxygen supply mainly to vital organs.

2. Vascular smooth muscles response:

   - The instant response of vascular smooth muscle to low oxygen is the dilation of peripheral vessels and constriction of pulmonary vessels to shunt blood away from poorly oxygenated lung tissue.

3. Carotid and neuroepithelial bodies:

   - Airway neuroepithelial bodies sense changes in inspired oxygen. However, carotid bodies work by monitoring arterial oxygen levels. Both send feedback signals to the brain to modulate ventilation and various mechanism to maintain oxygen supply.

   - Carotid bodies are highly vascularized and found at the bifurcation of the common carotid arteries on both sides.

   - Neuroepithelial bodies are situated at the airway bifurcation.

5.2 Regulation of cellular metabolism

Cell thrives by maintaining a high level of ATP, which plays a crucial role in different parts of metabolic pathways. Cell death occurs when ATP production fails to meet the energy maintenance demands of ionic and osmotic equilibrium. ATP production depends on oxygen supply. Thus, hypoxia induces cell death [5].

Mitochondria represent the main target of hypoxia, as it is responsible for generating ATP, response to hypoxia is by reallocation of cellular energy between essential and non-essential AT demands process.

Regulation of Gene Expression:

Response to hypoxia is by:

1. Increase ventilation

2. Increase cardiac output

3. Switch from an aerobic to an anaerobic mechanism

4. Improve vascularization

5. Increase oxygen carrying capacity of the blood

These responses take place early in hypoxia and are regulated by modifying gene expression.

1. Pathological response of hypoxia [5]:

2. Cerebral ischemia: The brain has high oxygen consumption, around 20% of the whole-body consumption. Under normal physiological conditions, this demand is met by an increase in cerebral blood flow. Ischemia develops when this process can no longer maintain an adequate oxygen supply to the brain. The longer the hypoxia, the more brain areas are affected.

   It is found that the most vulnerable areas are the brainstem, hippocampus, and cerebral cortex.

3. Myocardial ischemia: A brief period of ischemia (<20 minutes) is reversible if reperfusion is obtained.

4. Tumor angiogenesis: Most tumors during the growth period develop in the area of low oxygen supply that may trigger the formation of new vessels to maintain the growth, which explains how some anti-cancer treatments work.

Symptoms and signs of hypoxemia:

1. Headache

2. Dyspnea

3. Tachycardia

4. Bluish discoloration of the peripheries.

5. Cough

6. Wheeze

7. Confusion

Symptoms and signs of hypercapnia:

1. Shallow breath

2. Altered consciousness

3. Headache (cerebral vasodilation)

4. Pounding pulse and Tachycardia

5. Flushed skin

6. Profuse sweating

7. Irritability

8. Fever

9. Fatigue or sleepiness

10. Tremor and seizures

6. Pulse oximetry

It is a non-invasive method to detect the oxygen content of the blood by placing a probe on the finger or earlobe [6].

Uses:

1. detection of/screening for hypoxemia

2. targeting oxygen therapy

3. routine monitoring during anesthesia

4. diagnostic (e.g., sleep apnea)

Limitation:

1. Presence of carboxyhemoglobin, methemoglobin, fetal hemoglobin, and sickling red cells

2. Surgical and imaging dyes: methylene blue, indocyanine green, and indigo carmine may cause falsely low saturation levels.

3. Nail polish/varnis

4. High ambient lights level (fluorescents, xenon lamp)

5. Motion artifact

6. Reduced pulse volume: hypotension, low cardiac output, vasoconstrictions, and hypothermia.

Pulse oximetry is not affected by the following:

1. Anemia

2. Jaundice

3. Skin pigmentation.

7. Conclusion

In conclusion, Respiratory insufficiency can be divided into two main categories: hypoxic type and hypercapnic type, both have different pathophysiological mechanisms to develop. Note most of type 1 respiratory failure (hypoxic) diseases can progress to type 2 respiratory (hypercapnic) if not treated urgently.

Hypoxia could be a result of V/Q mismatch, right-to-left shunt, or diffusion restriction. However, decreased minute ventilation increased dead space, and increased CO_2 production lead to the development of hypercapnia.

Pulse oximetry is a noninvasive way to monitor the oxygen content of blood, but it has certain limitations that need to be considered before completely relying on it.

Author details

Mohammed Mohammednoor
Internal Medicine Trainee, University Hospitals Plymouth NHS Trust, Plymouth, United Kingdom

*Address all correspondence to: mohammed.mohammednoor@nhs.net

References

[1] Stenhouse L, Horton-Szar D, Whiten S. Crash Course Anatomy. London: Elsevier Health Sciences UK; 2012

[2] Mandel J, Cockrill BA, Weinberger SE. Pulmonary anatomy and physiology: The basics. In: Weinberger SE, Cockrill BA, Mandel J, editors. Principles of Pulmonary Medicine. Seventh ed. Elsevier; 2019. pp. 1-18. ISBN 9780323523714

[3] Roussos C, Koutsoukou A. Respiratory failure. European Respiratory Journal. 2003;**22** (Supplement 47):1-4

[4] Sarkar M, Niranjan N, Banyal PK. Mechanisms of hypoxemia. Lung India. 2017;**34**(1):47-60. DOI: 10.4103/0970-2113.197116, Erratum in: Lung India. 2017;34(2):220

[5] Michiels C. Physiological and pathological responses to hypoxia. The American Journal of Pathology. 2004; **164**(6):1875-1882

[6] UK RC. Advanced Life Support. S.l.: Resuscitation Council UK; 2021

Section 2

Respiratory Failure in Obstructive Lung Disease

Chapter 2

Acute Respiratory Failure in Exacerbations of Bronchial Asthma

Eva Sánchez

Abstract

Asthma is defined as a chronic inflammatory disease of the respiratory tract in which various cells and inflammatory mediators are involved. It is characterized by remodeling of the airway wall. Multiple inflammatory mediators may be involved, including interleukins. Physiologically, acute asthma has an early component, with an acute bronchospastic aspect marked by smooth muscle bronchoconstriction and a later inflammatory component, resulting in airway swelling and edema. In the early stages of asthma, hypoxemic respiratory failure occurs. If the asthmatic crisis is maintained over time, it will produce a status of severe acute asthma (ASA), which is characterized by hypercapnic respiratory failure.

Keywords: airway resistance (Raw), functional residual capacity (FRC), ventilation/perfusion (V/Q), interleukins (IL), acute severe asthma (ASA)

1. Introduction

From a pragmatic point of view, asthma could be defined as a chronic inflammatory disease of the airways in which various cells and inflammatory mediators are involved, conditioned in part by genetic factors, which occurs with bronchial hyperreactivity (BHR). Acute asthma attacks can cause great variability in gas exchange, as can be seen by measuring both the pressures of oxygen and carbon dioxide (PaO_2 and $PaCO_2$) on an arterial blood gas analysis, the same which may remain within normal values or experience a slight variation up to values that reflect severe hypoxemia, accompanied or not by hypercapnia.

2. Concept

Asthma is a chronic inflammatory disease in the airways. This state of chronic inflammation causes bronchial *hyperresponsiveness*, which leads to the narrowing of the conductive airways with airflow obstruction, which can be reversible spontaneously or with treatment. Asthma is a syndrome that includes various clinical phenotypes that share similar clinical manifestations but of probably different etiologies. From a pragmatic point of view, it could be defined as a chronic inflammatory disease of the respiratory tract, in the pathogenesis of which various cells and inflammatory mediators are involved, conditioned in part by genetic factors and which occurs with bronchial hyperresponsiveness (BHR). In patients with asthma, during acute attacks, arterial oxygen and carbon dioxide (PaO_2 and $PaCO_2$) values can range from nearly normal or slightly abnormal to extremely altered, ultimately resulting in profound hypoxemia with or without hypercapnia [1, 2].

3. Pathogenesis

One of the main triggers for an acute asthma attack is exposure to an allergen, which in susceptible people causes inflammation of the respiratory airways. The inflammation is generally predominantly eosinophilic, although the involvement of other cells, such as T cells, neutrophils, and mast cells, has also been identified. Many inflammatory mediators are involved in this process, including interleukins (IL)-3, IL-4, IL-5, IL-6, IL-8, IL-10, and IL-13, leukotrienes, and granulocyte-macrophage colony-stimulating factors (GM-CSF). In cases of sudden-onset, as is often with near fatal asthma, the infiltration is usually predominantly neutrophilic.

From the physiological point of view, acute asthma has two components: an early acute aspect marked by bronchoconstriction that occurs at the smooth muscle level; this, bronchoconstriction is usually episodic (asthmatic crisis or exacerbation); and an inflammatory component that develops later and causes edema of the airways [3, 4].

3.1 Early bronchospastic response

This response develops within minutes after exposure to a certain allergen and is characterized by the degranulation of mast cells or mast cells. This degranulation causes the release of immunoreactive mediators, such as histamine, prostaglandins, leukotrienes, and proinflammatory cytokines. These mediators produce smooth muscle bronchoconstriction and can compromise any level of the tracheobronchial tree, mainly compromising the peripheral airway (less than 2 mm in diameter in an adult). Other alterations that are observed are increased capillary permeability, mucus secretion, and activation of neural reflexes. This early response is characterized by a good response to inhalation therapy with beta 2-agonists [5].

3.2 Later inflammatory response

It is currently known that the airway epithelium is not only a passive barrier but an essential part of the local immune response in the airways, bridging innate and adaptive immunity against various environmental insults [2]. The release of inflammatory mediators primes adhesion molecules on the airway epithelium and capillary endothelium, allowing inflammatory cells, such as eosinophils, neutrophils, and basophils, to adhere to the epithelium and endothelium, and subsequently migrate to the tissues of the respiratory tract. A key inflammatory cell in asthma is the eosinophil of which there are increased numbers both locally and systemically in individuals with asthma. Eosinophils release eosinophil cationic protein (ECP) and major basic protein (MBP), and both ECP and MBP can cause desquamation of the airway epithelium and expose nerve endings. This interaction promotes increased airway hyperresponsiveness in asthma. This inflammatory component can even manifest in individuals with a mild exacerbation of asthma.

Bronchospasm, mucus secretion, and edema produced in the peripheral airways increase airway resistance and obstruction, by causing, in addition to airway closure, mucous plugging, and impaired mucociliary clearance. It has been determined that airway obstruction does not occur uniformly in the different lung areas. Air trapping will lead to lung hyperinflation, ventilation/perfusion (V/Q) mismatch, and increased dead space. The lung will then inflate near the end of the inspiration on the lung compliance curve and, consequently, can have a variable degree of increase in the work of breathing.

Lung obstruction and hyperinflation, resulting from increased pulmonary and pleural pressures, together with increased mechanical forces of alveolar distension, lead to decreased alveolar perfusion. The formation of atelectasis, together with decreased perfusion, causes a V/Q imbalance in the lung units with the consequent hypoxemia and an increase in minute ventilation [5].

In this sensitization phase, inhaled allergens are captured by dendritic cells (DCs) and presented to naïve CD4+ T cells in the presence of coactivators, including epithelium-derived cytokines, which promote T helper cell activation and polarization of 2 (Th2) that produce IL-4, IL-5, and IL-13. These T2 cytokines are also produced by type 2 innate lymphoid cells (ILC2) and are prominent orchestrators of the allergic inflammatory cascade that occurs in asthma. IL-4 drives B cell isotype switching and the production of IgE, which binds to the high-affinity IgE receptor on mast cells. Re-exposure to allergens results in allergen-mediated IgE cross-linking, causing rapid activation and degranulation of mast cells. IL-5 promotes airway eosinophilia, IL-4, and IL-13 act directly on the airway epithelium to induce goblet cell metaplasia and mucus hypersecretion, and IL-13 mediates airway eosinophilia. Airway hyperresponsiveness through effects on airway smooth muscle cells [5].

3.3 Airway remodeling phenomenon

Asthma is characterized by remodeling of the airway wall: epithelial cell loss, goblet cell hyperplasia, airway smooth muscle hyperplasia and hypertrophy, and thickening of the basement membrane, with increased collagen deposition and increased vascular density.

The lesion-repair processes cause structural changes in the bronchial wall (fibrosis, hyperplasia and hypertrophy, denudation of the epithelium) that are an expression of the remodeling experienced by the asthmatic patient's airway and will be responsible for a particular phenotype that shows worse airway control of the clinical parameters and response to treatment [3, 6].

This remodeling begins in the early stages of asthma, and a correlation has been established between the thickness of the airway wall and the severity of the disease. The thickening, along with the effects of increased vasculature, favors airway narrowing, the main long-term complication of asthma [3, 6].

Below is the basement membrane, which can increase up to five times in some asthmatic patients. This thickening has an impact on the efficacy of treatment since it correlates with limited responsiveness to glucocorticoid treatment.

Further down, we enter the submucosa, which in asthmatic patients is characterized by a marked increase in the vasculature and an increased presence of eosinophils and mast cells. These vessels are more permeable, which leads to edema and inflammation of tissues. The vasculature may contribute to the pathology of asthma in several ways: First, this increased angiogenesis with more permeable vessels may cause tissue edema and thus narrow airways; second, the exudation of plasma can aggravate local inflammation and remodeling; and third, an increased blood supply provides the hyperplastic and hypertrophied smooth muscle cells with the nutrients and oxygen necessary for their maintenance [6].

Even further down, we find the smooth muscle cells, which are the effectors that determine the diameter of the airways, causing them to relax or constrict according to different stimuli. Bronchoconstriction is the most serious symptom of an asthma attack, and these cells are the main effectors. In asthma, these cells are characterized by hypersensitivity to low doses of stimuli and hyperreactivity that produce a bronchoconstrictor response. This increased smooth muscle mass is already present in asthmatic children and youth without any signs of eosinophilic inflammation, suggesting that it could be the cause, rather than the consequence, of disease progression [6].

3.4 Other factors: Microbiome, microbiota, and asthma

It is estimated that the intestinal microbiome (a community of microorganisms that occupies a particular environment and performs a function within a specific environment) contains 150 more genes than the human being and there is a constant interaction between the two that, under normal circumstances, can thrive *via* symbiosis. Circumstances such as the country of origin, the route of delivery (vaginal or by cesarean section), and the use of antibiotics or lactation (maternal or artificial) influence the establishment of the microbiota.

Although we have less knowledge about how infections by viruses or bacteria, which cause many of the exacerbations of chronic respiratory diseases, modify the respiratory microbiota, recent studies have revealed the relationship between infections by certain respiratory viruses in childhood and predisposition to asthma.

When compared to that of healthy subjects, the microbiota of patients with asthma has a higher bacterial load, especially of the genus Proteobacteria, and less diversity in their lower airways. Instead, the Firmicutes and Actinobacteria genera are more common in healthy subjects. There is a relationship between the microbiota and certain characteristics of asthma, such as disease severity or resistance to treatment, as well as bronchial hyperreactivity. In fact, some of the bacteria could potentiate the allergic response of the airway. Other cohort studies, with various platforms, have shown that resistance to corticosteroids could be related to changes in the microbiome of patients. Thus, it has been shown that corticosteroid-resistant patients have a higher load of proteobacteria, including Neisseria and Hemophilus, while members of the Bradyrhizobium and Fusobacterium families predominate in corticosensitive patients [7, 8].

4. Pathophysiology of acute asthma

Various phenomena can be observed in acute asthma, the most characteristic functional alteration of asthma being increased airway resistance (Raw), particularly those located in the periphery (<2 mm in diameter). The main factors that cause a decrease in its lumen are smooth muscle contraction, mucus hypersecretion, and wall thickening due to inflammation and/or remodeling. There are also two important factors that also favor the closure of the airway in asthma: the alteration of the surfactant produced by the protein exudate of the inflammatory process, which can also undergo degradation by eosinophilic enzymes; and decreased *transpulmonary pressure* (TP), also called elastic recoil pressure. Under normal conditions, at the end of a passive expiration, there is a balance between the tendency of the lung to collapse and that of the ribcage to expand. The decrease in elastic recoil is important because when traction is lost in areas of the peripheral airway, they tend to close prematurely at the end of expiration, causing classic air entrapment. The classic airway changes in asthma (bronchospasm, mucus hypersecretion, inflammation, and remodeling) are added to this tendency to premature collapse. Air entrapment is manifested by an increase in residual volume at the expense of a decrease in vital capacity.

When an asthma exacerbation occurs, the lung loses elasticity, that is, the decrease in TP is accentuated, causing the equilibrium point between the lung and the rib cage to be reached at higher volumes (increased functional residual capacity [FRC]), which implies that the patient may breathe the same tidal volume, but with more inflated lungs. During forced expiration, the premature closure of the airways causes air entrapment, that is, an increase in the residual volume. If the asthmatic exacerbation is severe, regional abnormalities in ventilation may become unbalanced with respect to blood perfusion, causing hypoxemia, likewise, increased work of breathing can lead to muscle fatigue, hypoventilation, and hypercapnia [4, 9].

4.1 Bronchial obstruction

The basic functional impairment in asthma is airflow obstruction caused by a decrease in the caliber of the airway, especially during expiration. Bronchial obstruction is a diffuse and heterogeneous phenomenon, resulting from a mixture of spasm-inflammation and mucous plugs, which causes a significant reduction in airflow (peak expiratory flow, PEF, maximum expired volume in the first second of forced expiration, and FEV1). Sometimes it is found that there are no such mucous plugs, which suggests that bronchospasm alone can cause mortality asphyxia.

Although during an exacerbation, obstruction can occur at any level of the tracheobronchial tree, the peripheral airway (less than 2 mm in diameter in an adult) seems to be the main site of obstruction. Other functional abnormalities may arise from this alteration, such as increased work of breathing, alteration of lung mechanics and lung volumes, imbalance of the ventilation/perfusion (V/Q) ratio, and compromised gas exchange.

Although bronchospasm is the most important phenomenon, it would be simplistic to reduce the problem to obstruction since it underestimates the consequences that this causes on the distribution of ventilation [4, 9, 10].

4.2 Dynamic hyperinflation due to pulmonary overdistension

In acute severe asthma (ASA), the increase in airway resistance prevents the respiratory system from reaching its end-expiratory resting volume or functional residual capacity (FRC), because exhalation is incomplete, and alveolar pressure remains positive at the end of expiration. Lung hyperinflation places the diaphragm at a mechanical disadvantage, which causes the appearance of progressive pulmonary overdistension, which in turn causes an increase in end-expiratory intra-alveolar pressure (intrinsic PEEP or auto-PEEP), which is known as dynamic lung hyperinflation.

The respiratory pattern that the patient adopts in response to this is what contributes to the appearance of this phenomenon. Tachypnea and active expiration further limit expiratory flow by shortening expiratory time and dynamic airway collapse, respectively. Consequently, the balance point of the respiratory system moves to a greater volume than that of the FRC, which implies a greater workload for the inspiratory muscles, placing them in a position of mechanical disadvantage due to an unfavorable muscle length-tension relationship.

In all acute states of bronchial asthma, the ventilation/perfusion ratio (V/Q) imbalance is the main mechanism of alteration of arterial gases, being the determining factor of the degree of hypoxemia. On the other hand, hypercapnia is attributable to V/Q imbalance, although alveolar hypoventilation due to fatigability and/or weakness of the respiratory muscles also play an important role [11, 12].

4.2.1 Dynamic hyperinflation: Predisposing factors

Factors that predispose to dynamic hyperinflation are reduced expiratory time and increased respiratory rate, tidal volume, or inspiratory time. The initial tachypnea achieves an increase in minute ventilation and hypocapnia. However, the increased minute ventilation in the setting of airflow obstruction leads to dynamic hyperinflation, that is, incomplete exhalation and air-trapping. If the exhalation is incomplete, the alveolar pressure remains positive at the end of expiration; this is termed auto-positive end-expiratory pressure (PEEP). Lung hyperinflation places the diaphragm at a mechanical disadvantage [12].

A randomized placebo-controlled trial, which included 32 asthma patients on inhaled glucocorticoid therapy, showing dynamic hyperinflation, defined by a ⩾10% reduction in inspiratory capacity measured by standardized metronome-paced tachypnea test, showed that treatment with systemic glucocorticoids partly reversed dynamic hyperinflation, suggesting that it is caused by inflammatory processes that affect the airway in asthmatic patients. It was also observed that this improvement was more marked within the group of patients who presented greater eosinophilia [11].

4.2.2 Hemodynamic impact

Dynamic hyperinflation leads to hemodynamic consequences that represent the deleterious effect that air trapping causes on intrathoracic blood volume and can lead to cardiac dynamics. Pulmonary hypertension, due to compression of the pulmonary vasculature, alters the compliance of the right ventricle and causes displacement of the septum toward the left ventricle (LV). This phenomenon, known as ventricular interdependence, adds to reduced venous return's effect on LV end-diastolic volume and leads to a drop in cardiac output. The paradoxical pulse then appears as an expression of cardiorespiratory interactions in the severe exacerbation of asthma.

5. Acute respiratory failure

In the early stages of asthma, hypoxemic respiratory failure (type I) occurs, which can be observed on arterial blood gas examination as a blood pressure of oxygen (PaO_2) less than 60 mm Hg together with a blood pressure of carbon dioxide ($PaCO_2$) abnormal or low. This is the most common form of respiratory failure that accompanies most acute lung diseases and is generally due to fluid filling or collapse of the alveolar units. The disease process that causes progressive airway obstruction results in decreased oxygen available in the distal airways for uptake through the pulmonary capillaries. Through hypoxic pulmonary vasoconstriction, the blood flow of these lung units decreases, but this decrease is of less magnitude than that observed in the availability of oxygen.

If the asthmatic crisis is maintained over time, it will produce a status of acute severe asthma or *Asthmatic Status* (ASA), which is characterized by hypercapnic respiratory failure (type II) caused by excessive CO_2 production or decreased effective alveolar ventilation and characterized by a $PaCO_2$ higher than 50 mm Hg. The pH depends on the bicarbonate level, which, in turn, depends on the duration of hypercapnia.

All asthmatic patients are susceptible and at risk of developing status asthmaticus, which is a life-threatening episode of asthma that is refractory to usual therapy. Recent studies report an increase in the severity and mortality associated with asthma. In the airways, inflammatory cell infiltration and activation and cytokine generation produce airway injury and edema, bronchoconstriction, and mucus plugging. The key pathophysiological consequence of severe airflow obstruction is dynamic hyperinflation. The resulting hypoxemia, tachypnea, together with increased metabolic demands on the muscles of respiration, may lead to respiratory muscle failure [12]. If this state is maintained over time, it can inevitably lead to death.

6. Conclusions

- The airway epithelium is the first line of defense against pathogenic environmental factors. Therefore, the airway epithelium plays an important role in initiating host defense and controlling immune responses in asthmatic patients.

- The key pathophysiological consequence of severe airflow obstruction is dynamic hyperinflation. Dynamic hyperinflation in asthmatic patients with increased eosinophilia has a better response to anti-inflammatory therapy and eosinophilic biologics.

- Near-fatal or fatal asthma is a catastrophic, devastating clinical condition that occurs despite an increased understanding of its pathophysiology and pathogenesis.

- The intestinal microbiota plays an important role in bronchial asthma. Compared to that of healthy subjects, the microbiota of patients with asthma presents a higher bacterial load, especially of the genus *Proteobacteria*, and less diversity in their lower respiratory tracts.

Author details

Eva Sánchez
JUAN PABLO II" Private Hospital, Chiclayo, Perú

*Address all correspondence to: evasan2015@gmail.com

References

[1] Moral VP et al. GEMA 4.0. Guidelines for Asthma Management. Archivos de Bronconeumología. 2015;**51**(Supl. 1):2-54

[2] Rodríguez E. Essential Guide to Non-invasive Mechanical Ventilation Methodology. Editorial Panamericana; 2010. pp. 199-202

[3] Calvén J, Ax E, Rådinger M. The airway epithelium, a central player in asthma pathogenesis, review. International Journal of Molecular Sciences. 2020;**21**:8907. DOI: 10.3390/ijms21238907

[4] Rossi A, Roussos C, editors. Acute severe asthma: Pathophysiology and pathobiology of gas exchange abnormalities. In: Series "Clinical Physiology in Respiratory Intensive Care". Eur Respir J. Number 16 in this Series. Vol. 10. 1997. pp. 1359-1371

[5] Saadeh CK. In: Oppenheimer JJ, editor. Status Asthmaticus Updated. Jun 17, 2020

[6] Keglowich LF, Borger P. The three A's in asthma – airway smooth muscle, airway remodeling and angiogénesis. The Open Respiratory Medicine Journal. 2015;**9**:70-80

[7] García-Rivero JL. The microbiome and asthma. Archivos de Bronconeumologia. 2020;**56**(1):1-2

[8] Frati F, Salvatori C, et al. Review: The role of the microbiome in asthma: The gut–lung axis. International Journal of Molecular Sciences. 2019;**20**:123

[9] Michael J. In: Mosenifar Z, editor. Morris Asthma. Updated. May 11 2022

[10] Focused Updates to the Asthma Management Guidelines. A report from the National Asthma Education and prevention program coordinating committee expert panel working group. The Journal of Allergy and Clinical Immunology. 2020;**146**(6):1217-1270. DOI: 10.1016/j.jaci.2020.10.003

[11] van der Meer A-N, de Jong K, Hoekstra-Kuik A, Bel EH, ten Brinke A. Targeting dynamic hyperinflation in moderate-to-severe asthma: A randomised controlled trial. ERJ Open Research. 2021;**7**:00738-02020

[12] Shapiro JM. Management of respiratory failure in status asthmaticus. American Journal of Respiratory Medicine. 2002;**1**(6):409-416

Chapter 3

Respiratory Support for Obstructive Syndromes

Alexey Gritsan

Abstract

This chapter will present data on the biomechanics of respiration and gas exchange in acute respiratory failure of obstructive etiology. This chapter delineates main general principles of respiratory support, including non-invasive ventilation, and "traditional" mechanical ventilation. The principles of choosing positive end-expiratory pressure (PEEP) depending on the auto-PEEP are substantiated. The most commonly used respiratory support parameters for obstructive acute respiratory failure are presented. It is argued that the volume control (VC) ventilation modality is preferable in patients with asthma, since in this regimen positive inspiratory pressure (PIP) and inspiratory plateau pressure (Pplat) can be directly controlled, in contrast to the pressure control (PC) ventilation modality. The main options for selecting the ventilation mode will be presented.

Keywords: COPD, bronchial asthma, respiratory support, ventilation graphics, obstructive pulmonary disease

1. Introduction

Chronic obstructive pulmonary disease and bronchial asthma exacerbation are manifested by severe respiratory failure, which requires various methods of respiratory therapy. To date, enough information has already been accumulated to develop clinical recommendations for respiratory support in these diseases. We believe that special attention should be paid to the biomechanics of respiration in obstructive pulmonary diseases, the algorithm (step by step) of respiratory support, and indications and contraindications for non-invasive ventilation of the lungs. The choice of parameters for conventional lung ventilation is presented within the framework of the concept of protective ventilation; all the main complexities of mechanical ventilation management are identified; as well as the principles of weaning the patient from the ventilator.

2. Biomechanics of respiration and gas exchange in acute respiratory failure of obstructive genesis

It is well known that, like other skeletal muscles, the respiratory muscles can work with a load of about 60% of their maximum power indefinitely and without fatigue.

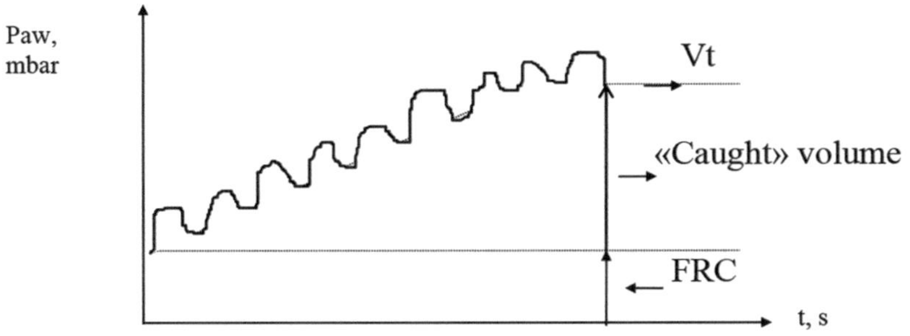

Figure 1.
Mechanism of formation of PEEPi, due to early expiratory closure of the airways (adapted from: Tuxen and Lane [1]).

Conceptually, if the load on the respiratory muscle's increases, or their maximum contractility decreases, then the respiratory muscles become fatigued, and eventually respiratory failure occurs. In bronchial asthma and chronic obstructive pulmonary disease (COPD), respiratory failure can occur against the background of the above factors (breathing demand and power (contractility) of the respiratory muscles).

Respiratory failure in bronchial asthma (BA) or obstructive pulmonary disease is associated with a sufficiently large increase in airway resistance (Raw) and increased work of breathing. As a rule, this is due to the presence of bronchospasm, the presence of a large amount of mucus in the tracheobronchial tree, inflammatory or fibrotic changes in the airways, or decreased lung compliance in emphysema.

The phenomenon of early expiratory airway closure that develops against this background leads to air entrapment (tidal volume (Vt) > exhaled tidal volume (Vte)), an increase in functional residual lung capacity (FRC), and, consequently, to overdistension of the alveoli with the formation of internal positive end-expiratory pressure (PEEPi) (**Figure 1**). The captured volume increases FRC and results in PEEPi (auto-PEEP). After each respiratory cycle, the "residual" volume increases. The consequence of these disorders is increased work of breathing, hypoxemia, and hypercapnia.

It is important to note that in bronchial asthma, these changes are usually acute (occuring during an exacerbation), while in COPD, the patient may be on the verge of respiratory muscle fatigue almost constantly, because of which even small changes in his somatic status can lead to respiratory failure.

Acute respiratory failure (ARF) of obstructive genesis is usually accompanied by overdistension of the lungs, which in most cases moves spontaneous breathing to a higher (less elastic) part of the volume/pressure curve (Vt/Paw), which inevitably leads to an increase in the elastic and resistive components of the work of breathing [2].

An increase in the work of breathing inevitably causes an increase in oxygen consumption and carbon dioxide production. Attempts to maintain the patient's $PaCO_2$ and pH at normal levels due to the more active work of the respiratory muscles lead to even greater production of CO_2.

Patients with COPD also have higher levels of dead space ventilation (up to 60–70% of Vt), which inevitably requires even higher minute ventilation and more work of the respiratory muscles to maintain pH at a safe level.

In patients with COPD, the activity of the respiratory center is also increased, but they are not capable of it in response to an additional load on the respiratory muscles.

The high stimulus manifests itself in high inspiratory flow rates with a corresponding increase in the work of breathing during the inspiratory phase. This failure of the respiratory center may add a central component to the development of respiratory failure.

As the demand for work of breathing increases, the ability of the respiratory muscles to do work is hampered by the obstructive process. Hyperdistention of the lungs is the single most significant mechanism in COPD, acting in such a way that the diaphragm enters a biomechanically unfavorable position in which it becomes unable to perform adequate work of breathing. Therefore, prevention and correction of lung hyperdistention are the two main goals of respiratory support in the management of patients with obstructive acute respiratory failure.

It is generally known that the tension developed by a contracting muscle is directly proportional to the length of the muscle at rest. In an emphysematous (inflated) chest, the diaphragm flattens and therefore geometrically shortens. The resulting shortening of the muscle fiber in the relaxation (rest) phase reduces the maximum level of contraction that can develop with diaphragmatic contraction.

The tension (T) that occurs in this case is inversely proportional to the speed of muscle contraction. When a patient with COPD or asthma and respiratory failure breathes rapidly and shallowly, the rate of diaphragmatic contraction increases, and maximum tension decreases. The amount of pressure that can be generated by a contracting diaphragm is determined by La Place's law:

$$P = 2T/R, \tag{1}$$

which means that the transdiaphragmatic pressure (P) for a given contraction is inversely proportional to the radius (R) of the curvature of the diaphragm. The increased radius of the flattened diaphragm significantly hinders its force of contraction.

As the overstretched diaphragm descends, its position in relation to the ribs becomes more horizontal, which prevents the ribs in the lower chest from participating in the inspiratory phase (Hoover's syndrome).

It is important to remember that diaphragmatic contractility is also affected by hypoxemia, hypercapnia, and acidosis.

The level of gas exchange disorders in obstructive ARF is characterized by hypercapnia with mild to moderate hypoxemia. Hypoxemia is caused by the following combination of factors:

1. violation of the ventilation–perfusion ratio (VA/Q)

2. intrapulmonary shunting of blood (Qs/Qt)

3. decrease in alveolar oxygen tension (PAO_2) due to hypoventilation of the alveoli.

As a rule, hypoxemia is easily corrected by a moderate increase in the oxygen fraction in the inhaled gas mixture.

The increase in $PaCO_2$ is due to decreased ventilation, increased carbon dioxide production, and increased dead space (Vd). Hypercapnia may further increase with the correction of hypoxemia through (Haldane), the essence of which is to raise the level of $PaCO_2$ with an increase in PaO_2 [3].

Thus, changes in the biomechanics of respiration and gas exchange during exacerbation of chronic obstructive pulmonary diseases and bronchial asthma, on which the tactics and strategy of respiratory support depend, are characterized by the following key criteria [4]:

1. increase in airway resistance (Raw)

2. increased work of breathing and flattening of the diaphragm

3. hyperextension of the lungs due to emphysema, the phenomenon of early expiratory airway closure, and a decrease in pulmonary-thoracic compliance (Clt) as a result

4. high Vd/Vt ratio

5. an increase in oxygen consumption and carbon dioxide production

6. hypercapnia and hypoxemia due to impaired VA/Q, Qs/Qt, and decreased PAO_2.

3. Basic principles of intensive care

The principles of intensive care in patients with obstructive acute respiratory failure depend on the severity of the ARF itself and are aimed at the following main goals:

1. elimination of bronchial obstruction (bronchodilators; corticosteroids; methods that facilitate the drainage of sputum from the tracheobronchial tree)

2. correction and maintenance of adequate gas exchange

3. maintaining adequate cardiac output against the background of PEEPi (infusion therapy, drugs for inotropic support of hemodynamics)

4. normalization of metabolism and acid–base state (ACS)

5. prevention of secondary bacterial infection (according to indications, the appointment of antibiotic therapy)

6. prevention of gastrointestinal bleeding against the background of the use of glucocorticosteroids (stress ulcer prophylaxis)

In this chapter, we will focus more on methods of correcting and maintaining adequate gas exchange using various respiratory support options.

4. Respiratory support

In the 80s, on an average, about 15–16% of patients with acute severe bronchial asthma required intubation and mechanical ventilation [5–7], while currently it is 2–4% on average [8, 9]. Bronchial asthma is a rather labile pathological process which may rapidly develop manifestations of acute respiratory failure requiring an immediate initiation of mechanical ventilation. However, in some cases, "aggressive" therapy aimed at eliminating bronchospasm, removing sputum from the tracheobronchial tree and/or mask (non-invasive) positive pressure ventilation can avoid intubation and mechanical ventilation.

Emergency intubation of a patient with bronchial asthma may become necessary in the following cases [9]:

1. the presence of cyanosis, $PaO_2 < 60$ mm Hg (despite oxygen therapy)

2. progressively increasing hypercapnia ($PaCO_2 > 55$ mm Hg) with altered sensorium with a GCS score of 9 or less

3. the presence of pathological pattern of breathing, silent chest, or respiratory arrest

4. the appearance of life-threatening cardiac arrhythmias or cardiac arrest.

4.1 Evidence of progressive exhaustion

At the same time, it should be remembered that the lack of response to drug therapy, severe metabolic acidosis, persistent hypoxemia, and patient anxiety can also be indications for patient intubation and respiratory support.

In patients with chronic obstructive pulmonary diseases, indications of mechanical ventilation include alveolar hypoventilation, a decrease in pulmonary-thoracic compliance, inadequate work of breathing, and unstable neuro-respiratory drive [10]. It should be remembered that patients with COPD, depending on the neuro-respiratory drive, are divided into two types: "Pink Puffer"—an almost normal respiratory drive and "normal" $PaCO_2$ and "Blue Bloaters"—a reduced respiratory drive and increased $PaCO_2$.

Tracheal intubation should be performed using a low-pressure cuffed endotracheal tube, and the largest possible endotracheal tube diameter should be used to reduce airway pressure levels. Orotracheal intubation is less comfortable for the patient, and there is a greater risk (compared to nasotracheal intubation) of unintentional extubation.

The main tasks of respiratory support in obstructive ARF are as follows:

1. maintaining alveolar ventilation

2. maintaining oxygenation at a sufficient level

3. ensuring the rest of the respiratory muscles, sufficient to recover from the state of fatigue that accompanies ARF.

However, it should be remembered that mechanical ventilation is a form of "physiological" support and should be carried out in combination with "aggressive" drug therapy for the underlying disease. Respiratory support should not exacerbate existing pathophysiological processes; it should be carried out in such a way as to minimize the occurrence of various complications. Withdrawal of respiratory support should not be attempted until the patient's underlying condition and comorbidities (if any) have improved.

4.2 Respiratory support algorithm

Correction and maintenance of gas exchange at various stages of intensive care in obstructive ARF is carried out using various types of mechanical ventilation modes: continuous mechanical ventilation (CMV), assist control mechanical ventilation (A/C MV), continuous positive pressure ventilation (CPPV), pressure support ventilation (PSV), intermittent mandatory ventilation/synchronized intermittent mandatory ventilation (IMV/SIMV), or continuous positive airway pressure (CPAP) or their analogues.

Because airway resistance (Raw) can change very quickly in this type of acute respiratory failure, pressure-controlled (PC) ventilation cannot guarantee adequate minute ventilation. Therefore, volume-controlled ventilation (VC, CMV) is preferred for most patients. A high level of Raw can lead to quite high values of peak inspiratory pressure (PIP), and therefore, a modern respirator is needed that can provide a given Vt at a PIP of at least 80 mbar. However, in some cases, when ventilation in VC (CMV) mode is unable to overcome high airway resistance, it may be necessary to switch to PC mode. In such a situation, dynamic control of the gas composition of the blood, SaO_2 and $PetCO_2$, is mandatory.

Typically, the starting mode of ventilation for patients with obstructive ARF is A/C MV. CMV is preferred for restless patients who have difficulty in comfortable synchronization with the ventilator and for patients with extremely high PIPs. Complete control of the patient's ventilation can be achieved through continuous sedation as well as the administration of muscle relaxants. Typically, CMV is continued until airway resistance and wheezing decrease. In patients with BA, improvement in the condition can be observed within a few hours, while in COPD this process may extend for several days.

Modes A/CMV or SIMV (or their equivalents) are more suitable for patients with comorbidities who are not prone to hyperventilation. However, when using these modes of respiratory support, the respiratory muscles perform part of the work of breathing, most of which can be spent to initiate mechanical (hardware) inspiration. At the same time, the fatigue of the respiratory muscles will persist, and the dependence on the respirator will be prolonged. Patients with extremely high respiratory drive may ventilate with A/CMV or SIMV at a high respiratory rate, which will inevitably lead to an increase in PEEPi and hemodynamic disturbances.

The respiratory support algorithm for obstructive ARF is presented as follows (**Figure 2**).

Based on this algorithm, the tactics and strategy of respiratory support are carried out in the following order.

Firstly, attention is given to oxygen inhalation or the so-called oxygen therapy. This technique is not a separate option for respiratory support; however, oxygen inhalations quite often accompany medical treatment of patients with COPD and BA in a hospital setting. One of the main goals of oxygen therapy is to achieve a satisfactory level of oxygenation ($PaO_2 \geq 60$ mmHg or $SaO_2 \geq 90\%$), which is quickly achieved in non-severe forms of obstructive ARF.

Since asthma has a low level of carbon dioxide retention, oxygen therapy is prescribed with medications (if there are no obvious contraindications). The starting level of oxygen concentration varies within 40–50% through a face mask or at a rate of 5 l/min through nasal cannulas. Subsequently, based on the data of the gas analysis of blood, the oxygen fraction in the inhaled gas mixture is corrected.

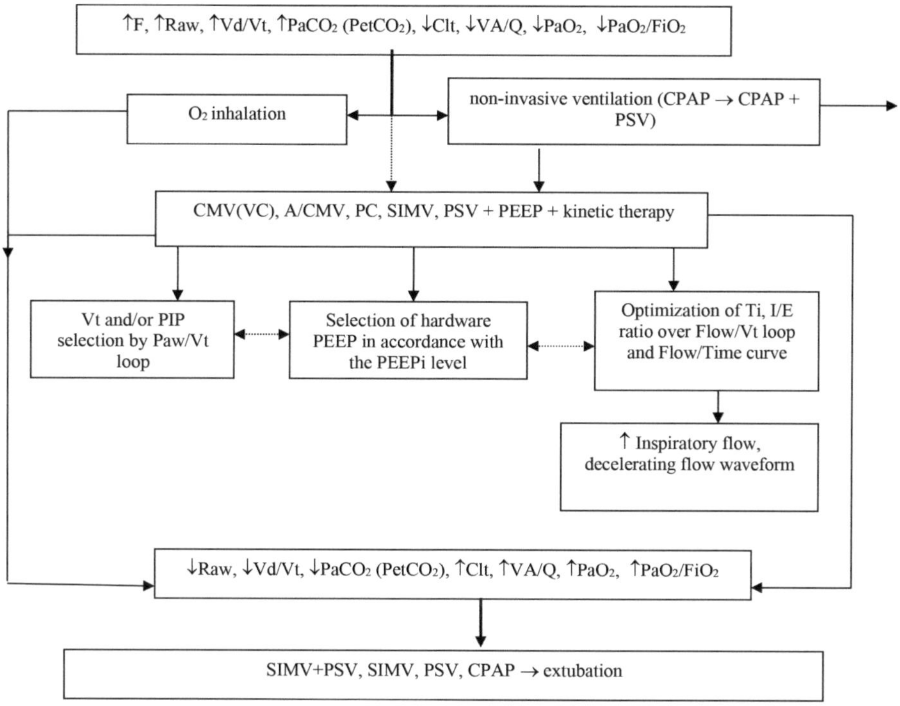

Figure 2.
Respiratory support algorithm for obstructive ARF.

At the same time, in most patients with COPD, the level of $PaCO_2$ in response to oxygen therapy will first increase by an average of 10–15, and then, it will stabilize. Therefore, a starting FiO_2 is set between 24 and 30% using a face mask or 3–4 L/min via nasal cannulas. At the same time, the $PaCO_2$ level should be carefully monitored (risk of carbon dioxide retention).

If, after 20–30 minutes of oxygen inhalation in a patient with obstructive ARF, the effectiveness of oxygen therapy is minimal or absent, and a decision should be made on the use of assisted ventilation.

When signs of ARF appear (increase in F, Raw, Vd/Vt, $PaCO_2$ ($PetCO_2$), decrease in Clt, V_A/Q, PaO_2, PaO_2/FiO_2), respiratory support begins with oxygen therapy or non-invasive ventilation (CPAP) followed by transition to CPAP + PSV. If NIV is ineffective, they switch to traditional mechanical ventilation in the following modes: CMV (VC), A/CMV, PC, SIMV, PSV + PEEP + kinetic therapy. Individual selection of Vt and/or PIP is carried out by the Paw/Vt loop, and the value of the hardware PEEP is selected in accordance with the level of PEEPi. Correction of Ti, I/E ratio is done on the Flow/Vt loop and flow/time curve by increasing the inspiratory flow rate and/or applying a decelerating flow waveform. With regression of signs of ARF (decrease in F, Raw, Vd/Vt, $PaCO_2$ ($PetCO_2$), increase in Clt, V_A/Q, PaO_2, PaO_2/FiO_2), respiratory support is withdrawn, followed by extubation. Detailed description is shown in the text below. Abbreviations: F—number of breaths, Raw —airway resistance, Vd/Vt—ratio of dead space ventilation to tidal volume, снижение Clt—pulmonary-thoracic compliance, V_A/Q—ventilation/perfusion ratio, CPAP—continuous positive airway pressure, PSV—pressure support ventilation,

CMV—continuous mechanical ventilation, VC—volume control, A/CMV—assisted CMV, PC—pressure control, SIMV—synchronized intermittent mandatory ventilation, PSV—pressure support ventilation, Vt—tidal volume, PIP—peak inspiratory pressure, Paw/Vt loop—tidal volume/airway pressure loop, PEEPi—internal positive end-expiratory pressure, Ti—inspiratory time, and I/E ratio—ratio of the phases of inhalation and exhalations.

4.3 Non-invasive respiratory support

Non-invasive respiratory support includes the actual non-invasive artificial ventilation of the lungs (through masks or helmets), as well as high-flow oxygenation through special nasal cannulas.

Non-invasive ventilation of the lungs (compared to "invasive" ventilation through an endotracheal tube and standard oxygen therapy) has several advantages and disadvantages.

The advantages of NIV over invasive ventilation are as follows:

1. absence of complications from tracheal intubation and prolonged need for the endotracheal tube
2. reduction in the frequency of nosocomial infections
3. reducing the need for medical sedation
4. the non-invasive nature of the procedure and its simplicity
5. the possibility of early mobilization of the patient
6. economic benefits.

The advantages of NIV over standard oxygen therapy through a face mask or nasal prongs are as follows:

1. providing positive end-expiratory pressure (PEEP) or continuous positive airway pressure (CPAP)
2. providing inspiratory pressure (Pinsp or inspiratory positive airway pressure (IPAP)) with inspiratory and expiratory trigger adjustment
3. adequate humidification and heating of the respiratory mixture.

The disadvantages of NIV are as follows:

1. the need for active cooperation of the patient with medical personnel
2. inability to apply high inspiratory and expiratory pressures
3. lack of direct access to the respiratory tract for oral hygiene
4. high risk of aerophagia

5. high risk of aspiration of the contents of the mouth and stomach

6. maceration and necrosis of the skin in places where the mask fits

7. hypoxemia when the mask is displaced

8. conjunctivitis

9. drying of the oropharynx and nasopharynx

10. nosebleed.

The use of non-invasive mechanical ventilation leads to an improvement in gas exchange, a decrease in the work of breathing, and an improvement in the prognosis compared with oxygen therapy alone (through a face mask or cannulas) in exacerbation of COPD (with the development of moderate respiratory acidosis ($7.35 > pH > 7.25$) and compensated ARF) [11–14].

The criterion for choosing non-invasive ventilation during exacerbation of COPD is the presence of respiratory acidosis, and not the level of hypercapnia: in the absence of respiratory acidosis, NIV has no advantages over standard oxygen therapy, at pH = 7.25–7.35 NIV should be used to prevent tracheal intubation, and when pH less than 7.20—as an alternative to mechanical ventilation [15–17].

In general, the main indications for the initiation of non-invasive respiratory support are the following clinical and laboratory criteria:

1. increase in the work of breathing (severe dyspnea at rest, respiratory rate > 25–30 resp./min, participation of accessory muscles, and abdominal paradox)

2. hypercapnia ($PaCO_2 > 45$ mm Hg and/or its progressive increase)

3. pH level < 7.35 and its progressive decrease

4. hypoxemia ($PaO_2 \leq 60$ mm Hg, $SaO_2 \leq 90\%$ with FiO2 = 0.4–0.5) and gas exchange disorders ($PaO_2/FiO_2 < 300$ mm Hg with FiO2 = 0.21, $Qs/Qt \geq 10\%$)

5. increase in airway resistance (Raw) from the norm by 1.5–2 times.

Non-invasive respiratory support should not be used in the following cases:

1. lack of spontaneous breathing (apnea)

2. unstable hemodynamics (hypotension, ischemia or myocardial infarction, life-threatening arrhythmias, and uncontrolled arterial hypertension)

3. inability to protect the respiratory tract (impaired coughing and swallowing) and a high risk of aspiration

4. excessive bronchial secretion

5. signs of impaired consciousness (excitation or depression of consciousness), inability of the patient to cooperate with medical personnel

6. facial trauma, burns, and anatomical disorders that prevent the installation of the mask

7. severe obesity

8. inability of the patient to remove the mask from the face in case of vomiting

9. active bleeding from the gastrointestinal tract

10. obstruction of the upper respiratory tract

11. discomfort from the mask

12. operations on the upper respiratory tract.

Tt is recommended to initiate non-invasive ventilation with a standard technique.

For non-invasive respiratory support, the PEEP (CPAP) mode with a pressure level of 5 to 10–12 mbar, or its combination with PSV (IPAP). Currently, NIV modes are practically no different from "invasive" ventilation modes (CPAP, CPAP + PS, pressure-controlled ventilation volume guaranteed (PCV-VG)), proportional auxiliary ventilation (proportional assist ventilation (PAV) and proportional pressure ventilation (PPV)), adaptive support ventilation (adaptive support ventilation (ASV)), in the settings of the device there is a setting for the backup mode of ventilation, and it is also possible to set both inspiratory and expiratory triggers. Randomized trials have not shown the benefits of any regimen for NIV [18–20].

The standard technique for conducting NIV is as follows:

- Set the value of PEEP 5 mbar

- Select the level of inspiratory pressure support (PS, IPAP) individually by stepwise increase from 5 to 8 mbar until reaching a tidal volume equal to 6–8 ml/kg of proper body weight (DMT) [calculation of DMT (kg) is carried out according to the following formulas: men = 50 + 0.91 × (height, cm—152.4), women = 45.5 + 0.91 × (height, cm −152.4)]. As a rule, this is achieved with a PS value of 10–16 cm of mbar.

- Set the minimum trigger sensitivity at which there is no auto-triggering (−1.5–2.0 mbar for pressure trigger, 2–3 L/min for flow trigger).

- Set the inspiratory fraction of oxygen in the inhaled gas mixture (FiO_2) to the minimum level that provides SpO_2 88–95%,

- Adjust the expiratory trigger sensitivity to improve synchronization with the ventilator (the standard setting of 25% is usually not suitable for patients with active inspiratory attempts and COPD, and such patients should set the sensitivity to 40–50%),

- Increase PEEP to 8–10 mbar in patients with SpO_2 less than 88% against the background of FiO_2 0.3 with an increase in PEEP tolerance.

High levels of PEEP/CPAP (>12 mbar) and/or PS (>20 mbar), despite a temporary improvement in oxygenation, lead to patient discomfort and reduced efficacy of NIV.

Reduction of dyspnea is usually achieved soon after an adequate ventilation regimen is established, while correction of hypercapnia and/or hypoxemia may take several hours.

In the first hours, assisted non-invasive ventilation of the lungs should be carried out continuously. Further, after a gradual decrease in respiratory support, it is possible to switch to NIV sessions for 3–6 hours a day until it is completely liberated.

It should be noted that NIV can also be carried out in volume, also equal to 6–8 ml/kg of proper body weight [21].

In the process of conducting NIV, it is necessary to monitor and evaluate the effectiveness of non-invasive ventilation of the lungs. If mask ventilation is ineffective, the patient should be intubated immediately, and "invasive" mechanical ventilation should be started.

Criteria for the ineffectiveness of NIV:

1. Inability of the patient to wear the mask due to discomfort or pain

2. Failure of mask ventilation to improve gas exchange or reduce dyspnea

3. The need for endotracheal intubation for secretion management and airway protection.

4. Hemodynamic instability

5. Myocardial ischemia or life-threatening arrhythmias

6. Impaired sensorium or delirium

7. Increase in F

8. Increasing the F/Vt ratio above 100

9. PaO_2/FiO_2 below 175 mm Hg one hour after the start of NIV

10. Increase in the $PaCO_2$.

4.4 Invasive (traditional) mechanical ventilation

In those cases when the patient's non-invasive ventilation is ineffective (or unavailable), invasive (traditional) ventilation is performed. This type of respiratory support is selected initially if there are indications for its implementation upon admission of the patient.

The main indications for the start of invasive mechanical ventilation are the following clinical and laboratory criteria:

1. ineffectiveness of non-invasive respiratory support

2. cyanosis, increased work of breathing (severe dyspnea at rest, respiratory rate > 35 resp./min, accessory muscle use, pathological rhythms of breathing, etc.)

3. severe hypercapnia ($PaCO_2$ > 55–60 mm Hg and/or its progressive increase)

4. severe acidosis (pH < 7.25 and its progressive decrease)

5. the presence of persistent and/or increasing hypoxemia ($PaO_2 \leq 50$ mm Hg, $SaO_2 \leq 85\%$ with $FiO_2 \geq 0.5$ or $PaO_2 < 35$ mm Hg when breathing atmospheric air) and gas exchange disorders ($PaO_2/FiO_2 \leq 200$ mm Hg, Qs/Qt ≥ 15%)

6. an increase in Raw from the norm by two times or more, and a decrease in Clt from the norm by 20–35%.

Initial modes (depending on the clinical situation) can be CMV (VC), PC, A/CMV, PSV, or SIMV (and their analogues). When using CMV, A/CMV, PC, and SIMV, it is most appropriate to use the following starting ventilation parameters: Vt = 6–8 ml/kg (with PC PIP level = 25–30 mbar), FiO_2 = 0.6, F = 80% of the age norm), I/E = 1:2, PEEP = 5 mbar, and flow = 35–40 l/min. If the PSV mode is selected, the selection of parameters is carried out similarly to the technique used for non-invasive PSV (see above).

A/CMV and PSV modes (or their analogues) require the installation of a trigger pressure on the respirator ((−1.5)–(−2.0) mbar) or flow (3–4 l/min).

Upon reaching, against the background of the above parameters of respiratory support, sufficient chest excursion, improvement in the conduction of respiratory sounds, $PaO_2 \geq 65$ mm Hg, SaO_2 = 93–95%, the oxygen concentration in the inhaled gas mixture is reduced to 0.45–0.3 under the control of SaO_2.

If the movements of the chest are limited, then it is necessary to increase Vt in steps by 30–50 ml (or PIP by 2–3 mbar) until a "normal" level of chest excursion is reached and evaluate the result.

While maintaining PaO_2 at a level of less than 60 mmHg at FiO_2 = 0.6, it is necessary to increase the level of PEEP in steps of 1–2 mbar until $PaO_2 \geq 65$ mm Hg, $SaO_2 \geq 92\%$.

Hypoxemia in obstructive ARF is usually a consequence of alteration of the ventilation–perfusion ratio and easily responds to a moderate increase in FiO_2. Setting FiO_2 = 30–45% is usually sufficient for SaO_2 > 90% or PaO_2 = 60–70 mmHg [2, 22]. High levels of oxygen concentration in the inhaled gas mixture may be necessary for patients with concomitant shunt-diffusive respiratory failure associated with acute respiratory distress syndrome, pulmonary edema, etc.

Further, after the improvement of oxygenation, hypercapnia, acidosis, the phenomenon of early expiratory closure of the airways and hyper distension of the lungs are corrected by optimizing the main parameters of respiratory support (Vt, MV, PEEP, Ti, I/E, and flow) in accordance with the concept of "safe" mechanical ventilation.

During selection of tidal volume, it is advisable to carry out based on the analysis of the Vt/Paw loop as follows: a stepwise increase or decrease in Vt by 20–30 ml until the "beak" appears or disappears on the volume/pressure loop (when ventilation is in PC mode, change the PIP value step by step by 1–2 mbar). That is, with the "optimal" Vt, there should not be a "beak" on the Vt/Paw loop.

Minute ventilation (MV) should be managed to correct the patient's respiratory acidosis over several hours by changing the number of machine breaths and/or Vt. It is important to note that pH is a much more important parameter than the $PaCO_2$ at which this pH is reached. Rapid correction of hypercapnia and acidosis can lead to post-hypercapnic metabolic alkalosis, hypokalemia, and hypophosphatemia.

In patients with COPD, one should not achieve a $PaCO_2$ value of 40 mm Hg and a pH of 7.40, since it is more physiological for them to maintain these indicators at the level that they have in remission. Slight hypercapnia and a moderate decrease in pH to 7.35–7.38 will help to avoid the occurrence of alkalosis and will not cause a decrease in neuro-respiratory drive or an increase in the severity of ARF during the transition to spontaneous breathing [2, 22].

4.4.1 *Internal positive end-expiratory pressure and selection of hardware positive end-expiratory pressure*

In everyday clinical practice, the most difficult is the selection of positive airway pressure, considering the level of internal positive end-expiratory pressure (PEEPi) [23].

PEEPi is the result of overstretching and high residual volume. PEEPi is detected in most patients with obstructive respiratory failure at levels often exceeding 10 mbar [24, 25]. If the expiratory time is insufficient, the high alveolar pressure will encourage exhalation to continue at the start of the next ventilatory breath. PEEPi has the same hemodynamic consequences as externally applied PEEP and can cause significant hypotension with tachycardia after just a few machine breaths in hyperventilated patients. Quickly disconnecting the patient from the ventilator helps identify the cause of hypotension, as blood pressure returns to normal immediately.

PEEPi also places additional stress on the respiratory muscles and contributes to the difficulty in withdrawing respiratory support. The value of auto-PEEP can be minimized by limiting the value of Vt and the frequency of machine breathing, as well as by lengthening the exhalation time and machine PEEP.

Clinical experience has shown that two techniques can be used to select the "optimal" level of PEEP and eliminate the phenomenon of early expiratory airway closure.

The essence of the first (the simplest) is to titrate the hardware PEEP (from the starting level) in steps of 1–2 mbar until the moment when, during auscultation of the lungs, the patient's exhalation becomes audible until the start of the next hardware breath.

The second technique is carried out under the control of $PaCO_2$ and $PetCO_2$ as follows:

1. The arithmetic difference between the partial tension of carbon dioxide in arterial blood and PetCO2 is determined, which in obstructive ARF varies within 8–15 mm Hg, with the norm of this difference being 4.5–6.0 mm Hg. That is, the utilization of carbon dioxide with exhaled air is insufficient.

2. The titration of the hardware PEEP begins by increasing it by 1 mbar every 5–7 min. When the level of PEEP becomes approximately equal to PEEPi, the utilization of CO_2 from the alveoli increases, which is accompanied by an

increase in $PetCO_2$ by an average of 15–25% of the initial level. An increase in $PetCO_2$ is observed within 20–40 min, followed by a decrease to 37–40 mm Hg.

In both cases, after selection, the value of the hardware PEEP varies within 9–14 mbar.

The criteria for obtaining an effect when using the methods are as follows: (1) a decrease in $PaCO_2$ by 25–35% of the initial level (according to the control gas analysis of blood taken 2–3 hours after the selection of PEEP); (2) spontaneous synchronization of the patient with the respirator, including after the abolition of sedation and/or muscle relaxation (if they were used).

4.4.2 Further steps of the respiratory support algorithm

The next step in "optimizing" the respiratory support parameters is the selection of the inspiratory time and the I/E ratio.

As previously stated, since lung hyper distension is always present in obstructive ARF, normalization of lung volume becomes the main goal. Functional residual capacity (FRC) depends on the ratio between the time needed to empty the lungs and the time to exhale. If the duration of the expiratory phase is insufficient, then the functional residual capacity of the lungs will exceed the normal FRC value. Each successive breath progressively increases lung volume until a new steady state is reached, typically 2–4 L above normal FRC [26, 27].

The time required to empty the lungs is a function of Raw and Clt and can be represented as a time constant (TC) that is the product of Raw and Clt. Since the time constant is the time required for exhalation from the lungs of 63% of the tidal volume that originally entered the lungs, the normal time constant for humans is about 0.42 s, while in COPD or bronchial asthma, these values are twice as high. Therefore, to avoid air entrapment, the expiratory time (Te) should be 3.5–4.0 TC, or 2.5–3 s [27, 28]. Large tidal volumes can also increase gas retention in the lungs.

Thus, to ensure sufficient expiratory time, Ti should be set as short as possible, and the I/E ratio should be set equal to 1: 2–1:4. At frequencies of 8–12 breaths/min, 4–6 s in each respiratory cycle will be available for exhalation, which in most cases is sufficient to ensure a full exhalation.

In addition to the empirical selection of inspiratory time and I/E ratio, it is advisable to use a graphical analysis of the flow/Vt loop and the flow/time curve (**Figure 3**). Increasing the length of expiration time by decreasing Ti and/or the number of machine respiratory cycles is carried out until a completely closed flow/Vt loop is obtained and the expiratory flow reaches the isoline on the flow/Vt curve at the end of inspiration.

Reducing the inspiratory time, of course, requires a change in the inspiratory flow rate (flow) to deliver a given tidal volume to the airways. That is, "large" Vt and short Ti require high flow rates.

However, one should not forget that the inspiratory flow delivered at a high level of airway resistance (which is present in patients with obstructive ARF) during ventilation in the CMV (VC) mode leads to an increase in peak inspiratory pressure (PIP). Because high PIP has long been suspected of causing pneumothorax and pneumomediastinum, it has been recommended that initial inspiratory flow rates are limited to 35–40 L/min. However, in practice, most of the peak inspiratory pressure is dissipated in the airways and is a less important factor in barotrauma than lung overdistension. Therefore, peak inspiratory flow rates reaching (if necessary for a particular patient) 80–100 l/min can be used [1, 5, 8, 27].

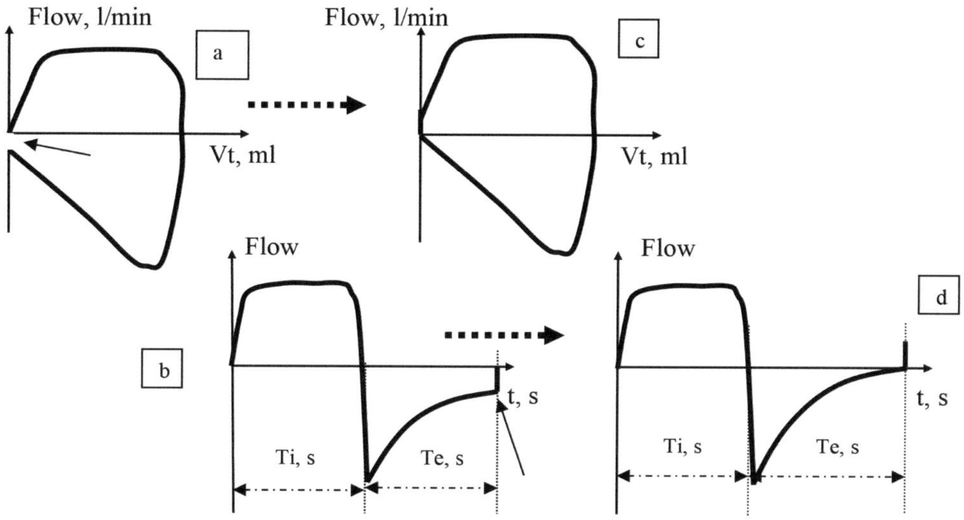

Figure 3.
Selection of inspiratory time (Ti) and exhalation time (Te)—According to the flow/Vt loop and the flow/t curve. The left side of the figure (a) shows an open flow/Vt loop (a) (shown by a solid arrow) and a flow/Vt curve (b) in which the expiratory flow to the beginning of the next breath (shown by a solid arrow), indicating insufficient time to ensure adequate exhalation (lung emptying). The right side of the figure shows the same graphs after adjusting Ti and expiratory time Te: The flow/Vt loop is closed (s), and the expiratory part of the flow/time curve reaches the isoline by the time the next breath begins (d).

If the technical capabilities of the respirator allow you to change the waveform of the inspiratory flow, then it is better to use a decelerating waveform, which leads to better gas exchange in the lungs compared to a constant or sinusoidal waveform of the inspiratory flow.

In general, based on this algorithm for the individual choice of mechanical ventilation options, it offers for everyday clinical practice the most used parameters of respiratory support for obstructive ARF, presented in **Table 1**.

Parameter	Values
Ventilation mode	VC
F, breath/min	8–14
Pplat, mbar	No more than 30
PEEP, mbar	5–15
I/E, ratio	1:3.0–1: 4.0
Ti, s	0.7–1.5
Te, s	4–5
Flow, l/min	Up to 80–100
Vt, ml/kgPBW	6–8
FiO_2 (0.21–1.0)	0.3–0.5 (until SaO_2 is 94%)

Table 1.
Most commonly used respiratory support parameters for obstructive acute respiratory failure (based on data from Laher and Buchanan [9]).

5. Difficulties in managing mechanical ventilation

Key issues related to the provision of mechanical ventilation in patients with acute and severe asthma and exacerbation of COPD include (1) methods for assessing pulmonary hyperinflation (described at the beginning of this chapter), (2) the effect of mechanical ventilation parameters on the severity of hyperinflation, and (3) the consequences and correction of hypercapnia [8].

It is known that the most common method for assessing hyperinflation is to measure the inspiratory plateau pressure (Pplat) and PEEPi during mechanical ventilation (**Figure 4**).

It should be remembered that PEEPi in severe asthma is often in the range of 10 to 15 mbar (cm H_2O) but may be higher.

Hypercapnia is common with mechanical ventilation in patients with severe asthma. At the same time, the $PaCO_2$ level can reach 68 mm Hg, at a pH less than 7.2, and a minute ventilation of 9 l/min [8]. However, the term "permissive" hypercapnia may not be entirely accurate when applied to severe asthma. Since hypercapnia is a consequence of increased dead space ventilation, attempts to lower $PaCO_2$ by increasing minute ventilation will lead to increased hyperinflation and a further increase in physiological dead space.

Serious adverse effects of hypercapnia are rare. Of greatest concern is the effect on the central nervous and cardiovascular systems. Cerebral edema and subarachnoid

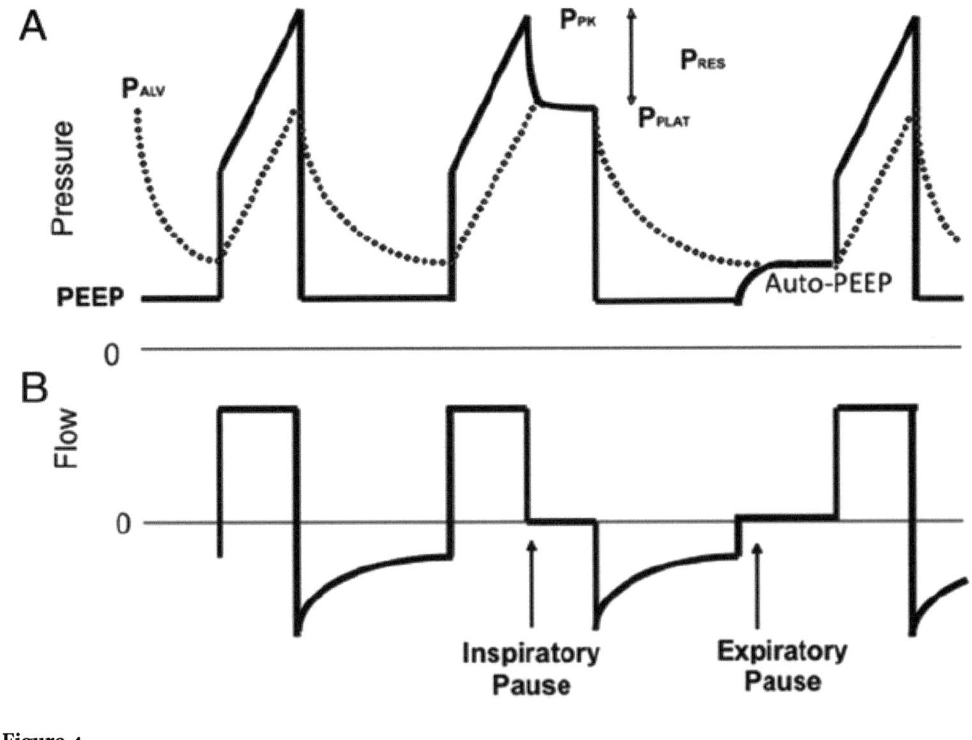

Figure 4.
Schematic representation of airway pressure (A) and flow (B) during mechanical ventilation. Note that the flow is maintained at the end of exhalation, indicating that the final exhalation of alveolar pressure exceeds circuit pressure (i.e., PEEPi is present). The dotted line represents Palv. Palv—Alveolar pressure; PEEP—Positive end-expiratory pressure; Ppk—Peak inspiratory pressure; Pplat—Inspiratory plateau pressure; Pres—Inspiratory airway resistance.

hemorrhage have been associated with hypercapnia but are rare. Acute hypercapnia increases cerebral blood flow and intracranial pressure, an effect of greatest concern in the setting of cerebral anoxia due to circulatory arrest prior to intubation. The cardiac effects of acute hypercapnia include a decrease in intracellular pH, which decreases contractility, but sympathetic activation more than compensates for this direct effect on cardiac contraction and cardiac output, which tend to increase. Arrhythmias associated with hypercapnia are not uncommon in the absence of underlying heart disease.

Alkaline agents may be considered when arterial pH is consistently less than 7.1. Unfortunately, sodium bicarbonate has a limitation in correcting respiratory acidosis. The CO_2 produced readily permeates cell membranes and can potentially lead to a significant decrease in intracellular pH during rapid infusions. In addition, even partial correction of severe respiratory acidosis may require several hundred milliequivalents of sodium bicarbonate. Therefore, in the absence of an urgent reason to correct the acidosis (e.g., severe arrhythmias, hyperkalemia, and unexplained hemodynamic instability), it may be prudent to withhold "alkaline therapy" and wait for the hypercapnia to decrease. Many patients experience a decrease in hypercapnia during the first 12 hours of intubation.

Another important point, especially for patients with asthma exacerbation, is the choice of ventilation mode.

The choice of ventilation mode must consider the degree of lower airway resistance and the presence of alveolar hyperinflation and "permissive" hypercapnia (as above). A high PIP, together with an increase in the pressure gradient of PIP to Pplat in the analysis of the graphical ventilation curves, indicates the presence of high resistance. PIP > 80–100 mbar is not an uncommon finding during mechanical ventilation in patients with severe asthma. Because the pathophysiology of asthma is not directly related to the alveoli, Pplat (which reflects lung compliance or alveolar pressure) is expected to be within normal limits (<20 mbar). Therefore, an increase in Pplat suggests the presence or increase in bronchospasm with an increase in hyperinflation or pneumothorax (**Figure 5**).

The VC mode is preferred in patients with asthma because PIP and Pplat can be directly controlled in this mode, in contrast to the PC mode. This should be kept in mind as long as Pplat is maintained below 30 mbar, even a very high PIP level (which is a sign of asthma) will not damage the alveoli (barotrauma).

When ventilating asthma patients, it is important to lower the upper pressure limit to a value that is higher than the patient's internal PIP. Failure to do so may result in fatal alveolar hypoventilation secondary to premature cessation of delivery of a given volume. This is better understood with the following example. If the upper pressure limit is set to 40 mbar in an asthmatic patient with severe bronchospasm, then tidal volume delivery will be terminated as soon as 40 mbar is reached. Because the anatomical dead space volume is one third (approximately 150 ml in an adult) of the normal volume (6 ml/kg), alveolar hypoventilation will occur. Therefore, the upper pressure limit should be set above the PIP (> 80 mbar in this hypothetical scenario) to prevent fatal alveolar hypoventilation. With a sudden improvement in bronchospasm (and a decrease in PIP), the patient will continue to receive the target tidal volume without an increase in alveolar pressure (**Figure 6**).

In contrast, PIP and Pplat cannot be controlled in a given pressure ventilation mode. Therefore, the patient will only receive adequate tidal volumes in this mode if the pressure limit as well as the set pressure is maintained above the internal airway pressure. With fluctuations in the degree of bronchospasm and associated changes in airway pressure, which can be sudden, there is a risk of either creating extremely high

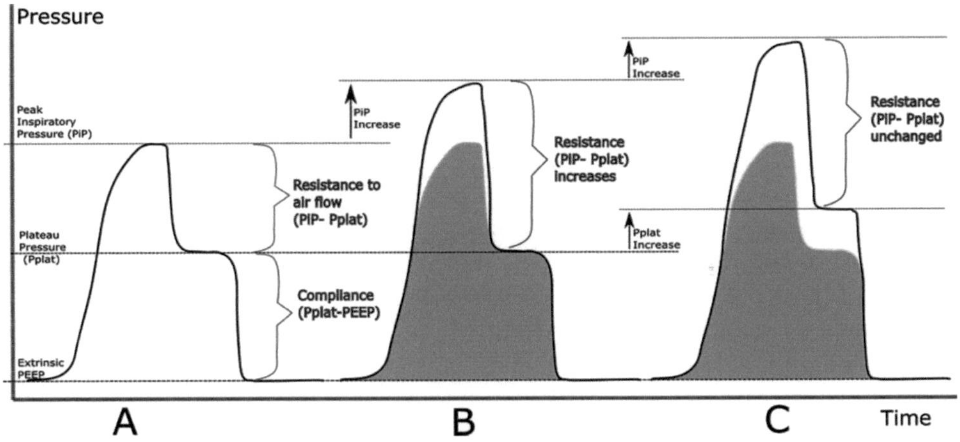

Figure 5.
Interpretation of the paw/time VC pressure–time curve in patients with asthma. A, Normal shape curve. B. Paw/time shape changes secondary to bronchospasm without hyperinflation. Note the increase in both PIP and PIP-Pplat gradient. Since Pplat remains the same as in A, this means an increase in airway resistance only in the absence of gas retention, since there is no change consistent with that in A. C. Changes in paw-time shape, indicating either (1) bronchospasm with gas retention or (2) pneumothorax. Note the same degree of increase in both PIP and Pplat. Since the PIP-Pplat gradient remains the same as in B, no further increase in the degree of bronchospasm occurs (shaded area, normal paw/time form). (Modified from Laher and Buchanan [9]).

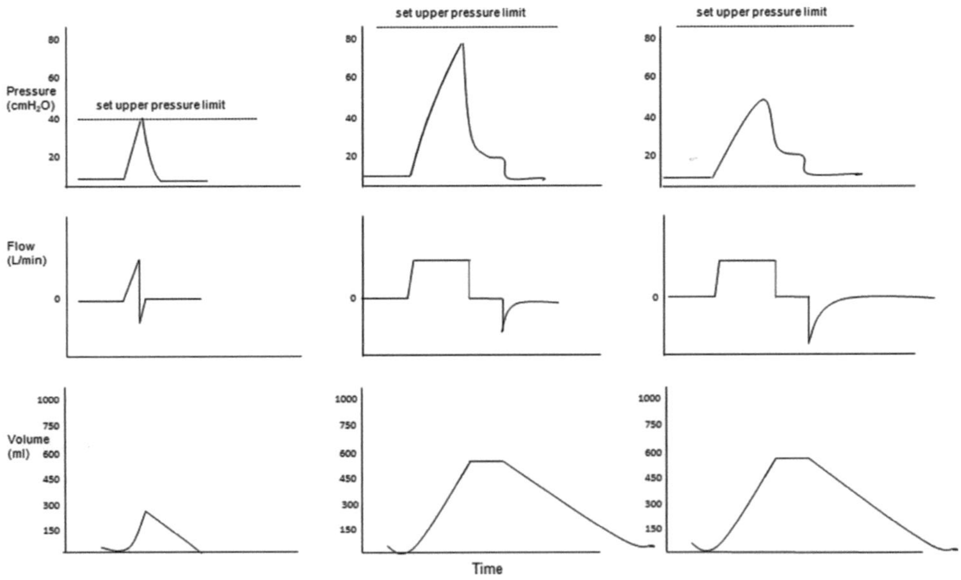

Figure 6.
Ventilate asthma patients using VC (recommended). Left: Patient with severe bronchospasm and PIP = 80 mbar. The upper pressure limit was set too low at 40 mbar; consequently, inhalation stops prematurely. Note the low tidal volume of 270 ml resulting in alveolar hypoventilation. Middle: Same patient with severe bronchospasm and PIP—80 cm mbar. The upper pressure limit is now correctly set to over 80 cm H_2O, with the patient now receiving an adequate tidal volume > 450 ml. Note that despite the high PIP (80 mbar), the plateau pressure is 20 mbar, which is within the recommended safe pressure limits. Right: Same patient with sudden improvement in bronchospasm (PIP—50 mbar). Although the upper pressure limit remains unchanged at >80 mbar, delivered tidal volume and plateau pressure remain unchanged at >450 ml and 20 mbar, respectively. (Modified from Laher and Buchanan [9]).

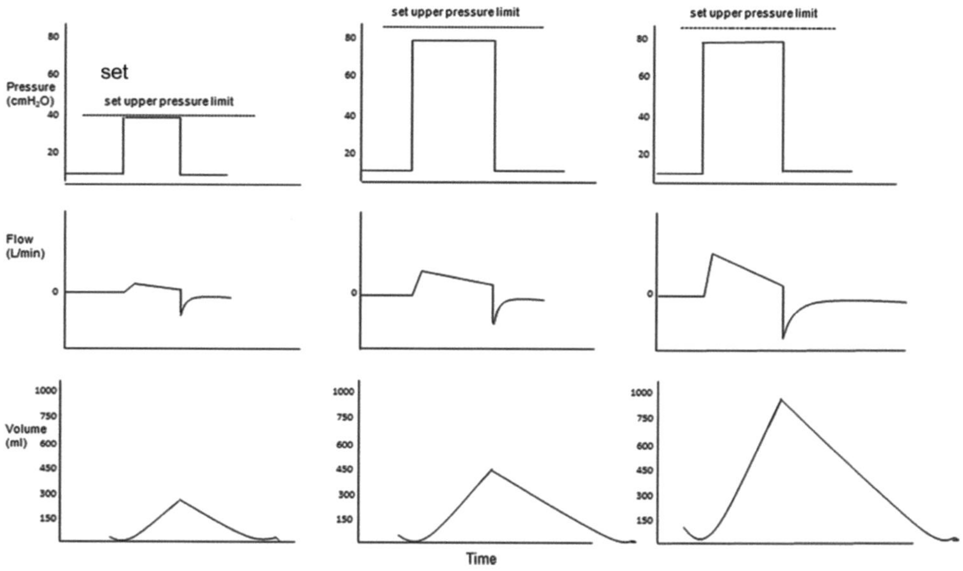

Figure 7.
Ventilate asthma patients using PC mode (not recommended). Left: Patient with severe bronchospasm and PIP—80 mbar. The upper pressure limit was set too low at 40 mbar, allowing only a tidal volume of 270 ml, resulting in alveolar hypoventilation. Middle: Same patient with severe bronchospasm and PIP—80 mbar. To achieve an adequate tidal volume > 450 ml, pressure control was set to 80 mbar, and the upper pressure limit was set to >80 mbar. Note that in this mode the plateau pressure cannot be determined; therefore, potential causes of high plateau pressure in an asthmatic patient (pneumothorax or gas retention) cannot be easily suspected in this mode. Right: Same patient with sudden improvement in bronchospasm (PIP—50 mbar) and established pressure control >80 mbar. Due to the sudden drop in airway pressure, the tidal volume (controlled by the 80 mbar pressure regulator) is now dangerously high (1000 ml), increasing the risk of barotrauma and pneumothorax. (Modified from Laher and Buchanan [9]).

and harmful or unacceptably low tidal volumes that may go unnoticed if alarm limits are not meticulously set and the patient is not under close supervision.

For example, if the above patient has severe bronchospasm and an underlying PIP (airway pressure) of 80 mbar, the patient will only receive adequate tidal volumes if an upper pressure limit as well as a pressure control/pressure maintenance level has been set >80 mbar. In case of worsening of bronchospasm, when PIP is increased (e.g., 90 mbar), the patient receives suboptimal tidal volumes, while if bronchospasm is suddenly eliminated (and PIP decreases), the patient is at risk of receiving extremely high and dangerous tidal volumes (**Figure** 7).

6. Weaning of respiratory support

If the underlying obstructive process is amenable to drug therapy, withdrawal of respiratory support and restoration of spontaneous breathing may be considered.

The patient's respiratory mechanics should be significantly improved by reducing expiratory time, dyspnea, reducing airway resistance and PEEPi, and increasing pulmonary-thoracic compliance. Sufficient oxygenation must be maintained at FiO_2 less than 40%.

Patients with asthma may be ready to withdraw within hours, while patients with COPD may not be ready for several weeks. Once the decision to initiate withdrawal has been made, all sedation and muscle relaxation should be discontinued.

With obstructive ARF, it is advisable to use the following additional criteria to make a decision on weaning a patient: (1) a decrease in peak inspiratory pressure to 17–20 mbar up to 8–11 mbar, PEEP up to 4–7 mbar; (2) improvement in the biomechanics of respiration (reduction of Raw to 6–9 mbar/l/s) and gas exchange ($SaO_2 > 93–94\%$, $PaO_2 \geq 80$ mm Hg, $PaCO_2 \leq 40–44$ mm Hg at $FiO_2 < 0.35$) [4].

One should draw attention to the fact that when canceling respiratory support, it is necessary to strive to optimize the response of the respirator to the patient's inspiratory effort, following the following rules:

1. Gradual (reasonable) decrease in the sensitivity of the trigger (from the maximum sensitivity of the triggering threshold equal to (−1)–(−1.5) mbar to −3 mbar)

2. The inspiratory and expiratory times set on the respirator should be as close as possible to the patient's respiratory pattern.

3. The flow rate of the gas mixture created by the respirator (both basic and inspiratory) must correspond to the needs of the patient.

To stop respiratory support in patients with regression of ARF, SIMV and BIPAP modes have been used since the advent of microprocessor ventilators, gradually reducing the number of machine breaths, PSV mode, and breathing through a T-shaped tube.

Several subsequent multicenter randomized controlled trials demonstrated the benefit of the spontaneous breathing test using the PSV regimen with pressure support of 7–8 mbar. Over the spontaneous T-tube test and the superiority of both methods over SIMV weaning in duration of ventilator weaning and failure rate [29–31].

The largest and methodologically well-designed study demonstrated a higher rate of successful weaning from mechanical ventilation using a 30-minute spontaneous breathing test with a support pressure of 8 mbar compared with a simple 2-hour T-tube spontaneous breathing test (without pressure support) [29].

Currently, to assess weaning from respiratory support, a spontaneous breathing test (SBT) is recommended for 30 minutes with a small level of pressure support to compensate for the work of breathing to overcome the resistance of the tube [29]:

1. Set CPAP/PEEP mode ≤ mbar. With PS ≤ 8 mbar.

2. Within 30 minutes, assess for intolerance to SBT:

    a. excitation or depression of consciousness—A score on the Glasgow coma scale of 13 points or less,

    b. $SpO_2 < 90\%$,

    c. RR >35 per minute,

    d. Tobin index <70,

    e. HR > 140 per minute or more than 20% of baseline or the appearance of arrhythmia,

f. decrease in blood pressure below 90 mm Hg. or more than 20% higher than the original,

g. participation in breathing of auxiliary muscles,

h. paradoxical movements of the anterior abdominal wall during breathing,

i. profuse sweating.

3. If the 30-minute spontaneous breathing test is tolerated, consideration should be given to disconnection from the ventilator and/or extubation.

4. In case of test intolerance, it is necessary to return to the previous ventilation parameters.

We pay attention to the following factors:

1. with all options for canceling mechanical ventilation during its implementation, it is necessary to maintain $PaO_2 > 60$ mm Hg, pH ≥ 7.35 at $FiO_2 \leq 0.4$

2. after extubation in some patients (especially with a long period of mechanical ventilation), it is advisable to consider using non-invasive respiratory support as a bridge.

In cases where it is difficult to wean from respiratory support in this category of patients, it is possible to use a semi-sitting position at an angle of 45° to reduce the level of PEEPi and reduce the load on the respiratory muscles [32].

7. Conclusion

In general, provision of respiratory support in patients with obstructive ARF against the background of COPD and BA requires the physician to both understand the main pathophysiological processes of the occurrence of ARF and a certain patience in the selection of respirator settings due to dynamic changes in the mechanical properties of lungs during therapy.

Conflict of interest

The authors declare no conflict of interest.

Author details

Alexey Gritsan
Department of Anesthesiology and Intensive Care, V.F. Voino-Yasenetsky Krasnoyarsk State Medical University, Krasnoyarsk, Russia

Address all correspondence to: gritsan67@mail.ru

References

[1] Tuxen DV, Lane S. The effects of ventilatory pattern on hyperinflation, airway pressures, and circulation in mechanical ventilation of patients with severe air-flow obstruction. The American Review of Respiratory Disease. 1987;**136**(4):872-879. DOI: 10.1164/ajrccm/136.4.872

[2] Honig EG. Chronic obstructive pulmonary disease and asthma. In: Perel A, Stock MC, editors. Mechanical Ventilatory Support. Baltimore: Williams & Wilkins; 1992. pp. 227-246

[3] Aubier M, Murciano D, Milic-Emili J, Touaty E, Daghfous J, Pariente R, et al. Effects of the administration of O2 on ventilation and blood gases in patients with chronic obstructive pulmonary disease during acute respiratory failure. The American Review of Respiratory Disease. 1980;**122**(5):747-754. DOI: 10.1164/arrd.1980.122.5.747

[4] Gritsan AI, Kolesnichenko AP, Lebedinsky KM, Kirov MY, Nikolaenko EM. Recommendations for respiratory support during exacerbation of chronic obstructive pulmonary disease and bronchial asthma. In: Collection of Recommendations for Respiratory Support. Krasnoyarsk: KrasSMU; 2009. pp. 117-132

[5] Higgins B, Greening AP, Crompton GK. Assisted ventilation in severe acute asthma. Thorax. 1986; **41**(6):464-467. DOI: 10.1136/thx.41.6.464

[6] Luksza AR, Smith P, Coakley J, Gordan IJ, Atherton ST. Acute severe asthma treated by mechanical ventilation: 10 years' experience from a district general hospital. Thorax. 1986; **41**(6):459-463. DOI: 10.1136/thx.41.6.459

[7] Dales RE, Munt PW. Use of mechanical ventilation in adults with severe asthma. Canadian Medical Association Journal. 1984;**130**(4): 391-395. PMID: 6362813; PMCID: PMC1876100

[8] Leatherman J. Mechanical ventilation for severe asthma. Chest. 2015;**147**(6): 1671-1680. DOI: 10.1378/chest.14-1733

[9] Laher AE, Buchanan SK. Mechanically ventilating the severe asthmatic. Journal of Intensive Care Medicine. 2018;**33**(9):491-501. DOI: 10.1177/0885066617740079

[10] Muir JF, Levi-Valensi P. When should patients with COPD be ventilated? European Journal of Respiratory Diseases. 1987;**70**(3): 135-139. PMID: 3569443

[11] Zabolotskikh IB, Gritsan AI, Kirov M.Yu., Lebedinsky KM, Mazurok VF, Trembach NV perioperative management of patients with concomitant respiratory failure. Russian FAR recommendations. Annals of Intensive Care. 2012(4):67-78

[12] Plant PK, Owen JL, Elliott MW. Early use of non-invasive ventilation for acute exacerbations of chronic obstructive pulmonary disease on general respiratory wards: A multicentre randomised controlled trial. Lancet. 2000;**355**(9219):1931-1935. DOI: 10.1016/s0140-6736(00)02323-0

[13] Girou E, Schortgen F, Delclaux C, Brun-Buisson C, Blot F, Lefort Y, et al. Association of noninvasive ventilation with nosocomial infections and survival in critically ill patients. Journal of the American Medical Association. 2000; **284**(18):2361-2367. DOI: 10.1001/jama.284.18.2361

[14] Girou E, Brun-Buisson C, Taillé S, Lemaire F, Brochard L. Secular trends in nosocomial infections and mortality associated with noninvasive ventilation in patients with exacerbation of COPD and pulmonary edema. Journal of the American Medical Association. 2003; **290**(22):2985-2991. DOI: 10.1001/jama.290.22.2985

[15] Keenan SP, Powers CE, McCormack DG. Noninvasive positive-pressure ventilation in patients with milder chronic obstructive pulmonary disease exacerbations: A randomized controlled trial. Respiratory Care. 2005; **50**(5):610-616. PMID: 15871754

[16] Barbé F, Togores B, Rubí M, Pons S, Maimó A, Agustí AG. Noninvasive ventilatory support does not facilitate recovery from acute respiratory failure in chronic obstructive pulmonary disease. The European Respiratory Journal. 1996;**9**(6):1240-1245. DOI: 10.1183/09031936.96.09061240

[17] Jurjević M, Matić I, Sakić-Zdravcević K, Sakić S, Danić D, Buković D. Mechanical ventilation in chronic obstructive pulmonary disease patients, noninvasive vs. invasive method (randomized prospective study). Collegium Antropologicum. 2009;**33**(3):791-797. PMID: 19860105

[18] Briones Claudett KH, Briones Claudett M, Chung Sang Wong M, Nuques Martinez A, Soto Espinoza R, Montalvo M, et al. Noninvasive mechanical ventilation with average volume assured pressure support (AVAPS) in patients with chronic obstructive pulmonary disease and hypercapnic encephalopathy. BMC Pulmonary Medicine. 2013;**13**:12. DOI: 10.1186/1471-2466-13-12

[19] Ankjærgaard KL, Tønnesen P, Laursen LC, Hansen EF, Andreassen HF, Wilcke JT. Home non invasive ventilation (NIV) treatment for COPD patients with a history of NIV-treated exacerbation; a randomized, controlled, multi-center study. BMC Pulmonary Medicine. 2016;**16**:32. DOI: 10.1186/s12890-016-0184-6

[20] Gantzhorn EK, Prior TS, Hilberg O. Long-term non-invasive ventilation for stable chronic hypercapnic COPD. European Clinical Respiratory Journal. 2019;**6**(1):1644893. DOI: 10.1080/20018525.2019.1644893

[21] Oscroft NS, Chadwick R, Davies MG, Quinnell TG, Smith IE. Volume assured versus pressure preset non-invasive ventilation for compensated ventilatory failure in COPD. Respiratory Medicine. 2014; **108**(10):1508-1515. DOI: 10.1016/j.rmed.2014.07.010

[22] Lindenauer PK, Stefan MS, Shieh MS, Pekow PS, Rothberg MB, Hill NS. Hospital patterns of mechanical ventilation for patients with exacerbations of COPD. Annals of the American Thoracic Society. 2015;**12**(3): 402-409. DOI: 10.1513/AnnalsATS.201407-293OC

[23] Wright PE, Marini JJ, Bernard GR. In vitro versus in vivo comparison of endotracheal tube airflow resistance. The American Review of Respiratory Disease. 1989;**140**(1):10-16. DOI: 10.1164/ajrccm/140.1.10

[24] Broseghini C, Brandolese R, Poggi R, Polese G, Manzin E, Milic-Emili J, et al. Respiratory mechanics during the first day of mechanical ventilation in patients with pulmonary edema and chronic airway obstruction. The American Review of Respiratory Disease. 1988; **138**(2):355-361. DOI: 10.1164/ajrccm/138.2.355

[25] Rossi A, Gottfried SB, Higgs BD, Zocchi L, Grassino A, Milic-Emili J. Respiratory mechanics in mechanically ventilated patients with respiratory failure. Journal of Applied Physiology. 1985;**58**(6):1849-1858. DOI: 10.1152/jappl.1985.58.6.1849

[26] Kimball WR, Leith DE, Robins AG. Dynamic hyperinflation and ventilator dependence in chronic obstructive pulmonary disease. The American Review of Respiratory Disease. 1982; **126**(6):991-995. DOI: 10.1164/arrd.1982.126.6.991

[27] García Vicente E, Sandoval Almengor JC, Díaz Caballero LA, Salgado Campo JC. Ventilación mecánica invasiva en EPOC y asma [Invasive mechanical ventilation in COPD and asthma]. Medicina Intensiva. 2011;**35**(5): 288-298. Spanish. DOI: 10.1016/j.medin.2010.11.004

[28] Bergman NA. Intrapulmonary gas trapping during mechanical ventilation at rapid frequencies. Anesthesiology. 1972;**37**(6):626-633. DOI: 10.1097/00000542-197212000-00011

[29] Subirà C, Hernández G, Vázquez A, Rodríguez-García R, González-Castro A, García C, et al. Effect of pressure support vs T-piece ventilation strategies during spontaneous breathing trials on successful Extubation among patients receiving mechanical ventilation: A randomized clinical trial. Journal of the American Medical Association. 2019; **321**(22):2175-2182. DOI: 10.1001/jama.2019.7234

[30] Esteban A, Alía I, Gordo F, Fernández R, Solsona JF, Vallverdú I, et al. Extubation outcome after spontaneous breathing trials with T-tube or pressure support ventilation. The Spanish lung failure collaborative group. American Journal of Respiratory and Critical Care Medicine. 1997;**156**(2 Pt 1): 459-465. DOI: 10.1164/ajrccm.156.2.9610109

[31] Brochard L, Rauss A, Benito S, Conti G, Mancebo J, Rekik N, et al. Comparison of three methods of gradual withdrawal from ventilatory support during weaning from mechanical ventilation. American Journal of Respiratory and Critical Care Medicine. 1994;**150**(4):896-903. DOI: 10.1164/ajrccm.150.4.7921460

[32] Deye N, Lellouche F, Maggiore SM, Taillé S, Demoule A, L'Her E, et al. The semi-seated position slightly reduces the effort to breathe during difficult weaning. Intensive Care Medicine. 2013; **39**(1):85-92. DOI: 10.1007/s00134-012-2727-5

Section 3

Respiratory Failure in COVID-19

Chapter 4

Respiratory Failure in COVID-19 Condition

Olalekan Bukunmi Ogunro and Oluwaseun Ruth Olasehinde

Abstract

Respiratory failure, characterized as the unsuccessful maintenance of adequate gas exchange, is associated with abnormalities of arterial blood gas tensions. The coronavirus disease-2019 (COVID-19) is majorly a respiratory disease capable of causing infection caused by the newly discovered coronavirus (SARS-CoV-2) with a consequential effect on respiratory failure. Simply put, respiratory failure is the major clinical demonstration of COVID-19 and the frontline cause of the associated mortality. Respiratory failure instigated by COVID-19 has some clinical features in affected patients. Disorders of the respiratory neuromuscular, airway, pulmonary vesicles, and lung parenchyma all manifest in COVID-19. These features are heterogeneous and categorized into progressive respiratory distress and unique "silent hypoxemia" as two phenotypes. Knowing the exact phenotype in patients with COVID-19 has been of important clinical significance in seeking the right treatment strategies for treating respiratory failure. The chapter will, therefore, provide more insights into the pathophysiology, clinical attributes, pathogenesis, and treatment approach of respiratory failure in COVID-19 conditions, as well as evaluate any similarities and differences that may exist.

Keywords: COVID-19, respiratory insufficiency, breathing difficulty, ventilation, oxygenation, respiratory dysfunction, respiratory failure, SARS-CoV-2

1. Introduction

Breathing is an indispensable requirement in life. Ideally, in humans and all mammals, oxygen (O_2) from the air is breathed into the lungs, while carbon dioxide (CO_2) is breathed out as a waste product made by cells of the body. Oxygen utilization and carbon dioxide production are, therefore, essential to life. The proper function of tissues and organs requires adequate oxygen from the lungs into the blood. The respiratory system allows the entry of O_2 and the parting of CO_2 in the body. Accumulated carbon dioxide causes severe damage and injury to these tissues and organs and slows the rate of delivery of oxygen to the body.

Respiratory failure is a grave condition that makes breathing difficult without any aid and usually sets in when the lungs are unable to get adequate oxygen (hypoxic respiratory failure) into the blood or the difficulty of the lungs to get rid of carbon dioxide (ventilator failure) to meet metabolic requirements. Acute respiratory failure may be quick and happens without prior notice. In most cases, it is associated with breathing diseases/injuries such as pneumonia, stroke, opioid overdose, or even injury of the spinal cord or lungs.

Patients with respiratory issues can have illness from a family of viruses known as coronavirus. The term "corona" refers to the surface of the virus, which is coated in spikes like crowns. Examples of coronaviruses that infect humans include the common cold and severe acute respiratory syndrome (SARS). A new coronavirus known as severe acute respiratory syndrome coronavirus-2 (SARS-CoV-2) is the cause of the infectious disease known as coronavirus disease-2019 (COVID-19) [1, 2]. The coronavirus disease 2019 (COVID-19) pandemic is caused by the novel coronavirus regarded as severe acute respiratory syndrome coronavirus 2 (SARS-CoV-2). COVID-19 was identified initially in December 2019 in Wuhan, China, by several patients. Since then, COVID-19 has raised myriad global concerns [1]. One of the resultant effects of COVID-19 is lung damage with gradual declination may result in acute hypoxic respiratory failure and, in the worst scenario, results in acute respiratory distress syndrome (ARDS). Acute hypoxemic respiratory failure is a major clinical feature of COVID-19 during inflammation of the lungs. COVID-19-related respiratory failure has features of injury to the alveolar epithelium cells, while the endothelium cells may be less damaged [3].

Apart from meeting the Berlin definition of ARDS, COVID-19 has uniqueness in both pathological and pathophysiological characteristics, not limited to endothelial injury, pulmonary capillary hyperplasia, and extensive microthrombus [4]. COVID-19 can, therefore, be regarded as a preponderantly respiratory infectious disease with respiratory failure as the principal clinical outcome and the pre-eminent cause of mortality [5].

As in patients who battle with respiratory failure instigated by other means, heterogeneity of clinical features exists in persons with respiratory failure instigated by COVID-19. The gradually advancing respiratory distress and distinct silent hypoxemia are the two phenotypes. Recognition of the exact phenotypes in patients with COVID-19 will be of immense value for the best treatment options. In most cases recorded, respiratory failure due to COVID-19 develops very quickly because this disease affects the respiratory system primarily while damage to other organs may be secondary [6]. Since there is still no major cure treatment for COVID-19, it is therefore important that the key therapeutic intervention focuses on symptomatic treatment of respiratory failure. This chapter is focused on providing scientific insights into the epidemiology, pathophysiology, and clinical features of respiratory failure in COVID-19 conditions to help healthcare professionals manage patients with COVID-19.

2. Respiratory failure

The system for taking in oxygen and releasing carbon dioxide commences at the nose and mouth and goes through the airways and the lungs. Air usually comes in through the respiratory system via the nose and mouth and is then taken down the pharynx through the larynx. A cartilaginous structure known as epiglottis usually covers the entrance to the larynx. The epiglottis prevents food from getting into the airways by closing automatically during food intake [7].

Respiratory failure sets in when the respiratory system fails to meet the oxygen and ventilatory demands of an individual/patient. Respiratory failure, therefore, is a clinical term that defines the failure of the respiratory system to preserve its physiological role of gas exchange such that PaO2 maintained is not beyond 60 mmHg and/or PaCO2 greater than 50 mmHg. Respiratory failure happens when the breathing system cannot sustain enough levels of blood oxygen, as well as difficulties in eliminating carbon dioxide in the blood [8]. Respiratory failure can be a slow development with symptoms not limited to shortness of breath, distress in breathing, extreme tiredness, restlessness, and drowsiness (when the low oxygen level is low), as well as headaches, blurry sight, disarray, speedy breathing (carbon dioxide levels is high). In newborns, symptoms of respiratory failure may include inward pull of the ribs' muscles, speedy breath, nostrils broadening with the breath, grunting, and bluish skin and lips tone. Respiratory failure poses a serious threat to the lungs and other vital organs [9].

Diagnosis of respiratory failure may be determined by the blood levels of oxygen and carbon dioxide levels apart from a physical examination. Generally, factors such as the blood levels of oxygen and carbon dioxide, causative factors, and rate of development determine the symptoms associated with respiratory failure. Acute respiratory failure can result in a life-threatening emergency that necessitates additional oxygen through nasal tubes or a breathing-aided machine (ventilator) [10].

Factors such as age, environment, medical condition, lifestyle habits, or drugs increase the risk of respiratory failure. For instance, infants with neonatal respiratory distress because of the under-developed lung, certain lung birth defects, or

S/N	Circumstances	Conditions	Outcome
1	Difficulty in breathing	Weakness following collapsed airways and stroke	Blockage of the windpipe
2	Difficulty exhaling	Asthma condition and conditions of chronic obstructive pulmonary disease	Narrowing of airways; accumulation of mucus and narrowing of the airways
3	The difficulty of air entry to the lungs	Weak muscles, severe pains, airway blockage by mucus, fractured or broken ribs, and pneumothorax	respiratory failure
4	Retention of fluid in the lungs	Lack of oxygen passage from the air sacs into the blood makes it difficult for the blood's carbon dioxide to enter the air sacs to be exhaled	Accumulation of fluid in the lungs associated with the condition such as ARDS, pneumonia, drowning, heart failure, and head injury or trauma
5	Breathing muscles difficulties	Spinal cord trauma or condition of many diseases of the muscular system (occurring among members of a family) due to inadequate oxygen-rich blood in reaching the diaphragm and other breathing muscles or condition of cardiogenic shock and sepsis	Non-vitality and muscle wasting (muscular dystrophy)
6	Situations that affect the brain's control over breathing, usually when there is an overdose of drugs like an opioid overdose	High concentrations of carbon dioxide in the blood detected by the brain	Accumulation of carbon dioxide in the body while the concentration of oxygen fall

Table 1.
Circumstances, conditions, and the resultant effect of respiratory failure.

pulmonary hypertension are more vulnerable to respiratory failure, while aged persons with weak breathing muscles or with a common cold or allergies are more prone to respiratory failure [11]. Also, breathing lung irritants (such as dust, chemical fumes, dyes and paints, asbestos, aniline, or smoke) from the environment for a long period of time can lead to lung damage and pose a risk of severe lung diseases [12]. There is also more danger of respiratory failure with some medical conditions such as disorders of the muscles and nerve (like Guillain-Barre syndrome, amyotrophic lateral sclerosis, and myasthenia); diseases of the airways and lungs (cystic fibrosis, interstitial lung diseases, asthma, and COPD); congestive heart failure or pulmonary embolism; spinal cord or brain infections; meningitis; pneumonia; bronchiolitis; obstructed airway; chest or back injuries; severe scoliosis; and food or drug allergies [13, 14]. Moreover, life habits like smoking can instigate diseases of the lungs and potentiate vulnerability to respiratory failure. Indiscriminate alcohol or drugs affects the area of the brain that controls breathing by making breathing becomes slow and shallow and may ultimately give rise to acute respiratory failure. In addition, some sedatives used during surgery raise the risk of respiratory failure [15]. Respiratory failure may be a resultant effect of many factors described in **Table 1**.

Respiratory failure can be classified as hypoxemic (Type 1) and hypercapnic (Type 2). Hypercapnia often results from a failed respiratory, leading to PaCO2 greater than 50 mmHg. In the hypoxemic respiratory failure associated with COVID-19, ARDs, severe pneumonia, and edema, PaO2 is lesser than 60 mmHg with normal or subnormal PaCO2 [16].

3. Pathogenesis and pathology of ARDS-associated and non-associated COVID-19

In contrast to the conventional ARDS, the pathogen of COVID-19 is obvious; SARS-CoV-2 causes it, a beta-coronavirus that gains entry into the cells by binding the angiotensin-converting enzyme 2 (ACE2) receptor *via* the viral structural spike (S) protein. Alveoli (II) epithelial cells, small intestine, bronchia, vesicle, and numerous types of immune cells, such as macrophages, monocytes, and dendritic cells, all contain ACE2 receptors in varying degrees. As a result of attacking the lung immune cells, SARS-CoV-2 can cause a lower respiratory infection and trigger an inflammatory reaction [17].

Comparing COVID-19 to a typical case of ARDS, the pathophysiology is more complex and varied. Some patients with acute COVID-19 proceeded to well-known ARDS, although a sizable portion of these patients did not exhibit the "reduced lung capacity and impaired compliance" that are typical of classical ARDS. In contrast to how severe the hypoxemia is, their pulmonary compliance is almost normal. Additionally, intrapulmonary shunt, along with dead space ventilation, is the primary cause of ARDS-related hypoxemia [4, 18]. Hypoxemia caused by COVID-19 can be understood by dysfunctional hypoxic pulmonary vasoconstriction, which impairs lung perfusion regulation, and microthrombus of the lung alveoli, which simultaneously increases dead space and causes intrapulmonary shunt. Reports have shown that patients with COVID-19 experience hypoxemia for a variety of reasons, including vascular dysfunction, dead space, and intrapulmonary shunt [19].

Gattinoni et al. classified the COVID-19 phenotype as type H and type L. The following were the key L-type symptoms: (1) Low elastance, almost normal compliance, and nearly normal lung gas content are indicators of low elastance. (2) Low ventilation to perfusion ratio. (3) Lightweight lungs and (4) Limited lung recruitment. Although there is significant hypoxemia in these patients, respiratory compliance is beyond 50 ml/cm H2O. The lung is not very recruitable and contains a lot of gas. The main cause of severe hypoxia is the impaired ventilation-to-perfusion ratio [20].

High PEEP and prone positioning are used to increase oxygenation, but not by encouraging the enlargement of the collapsed alveolar region, but rather by

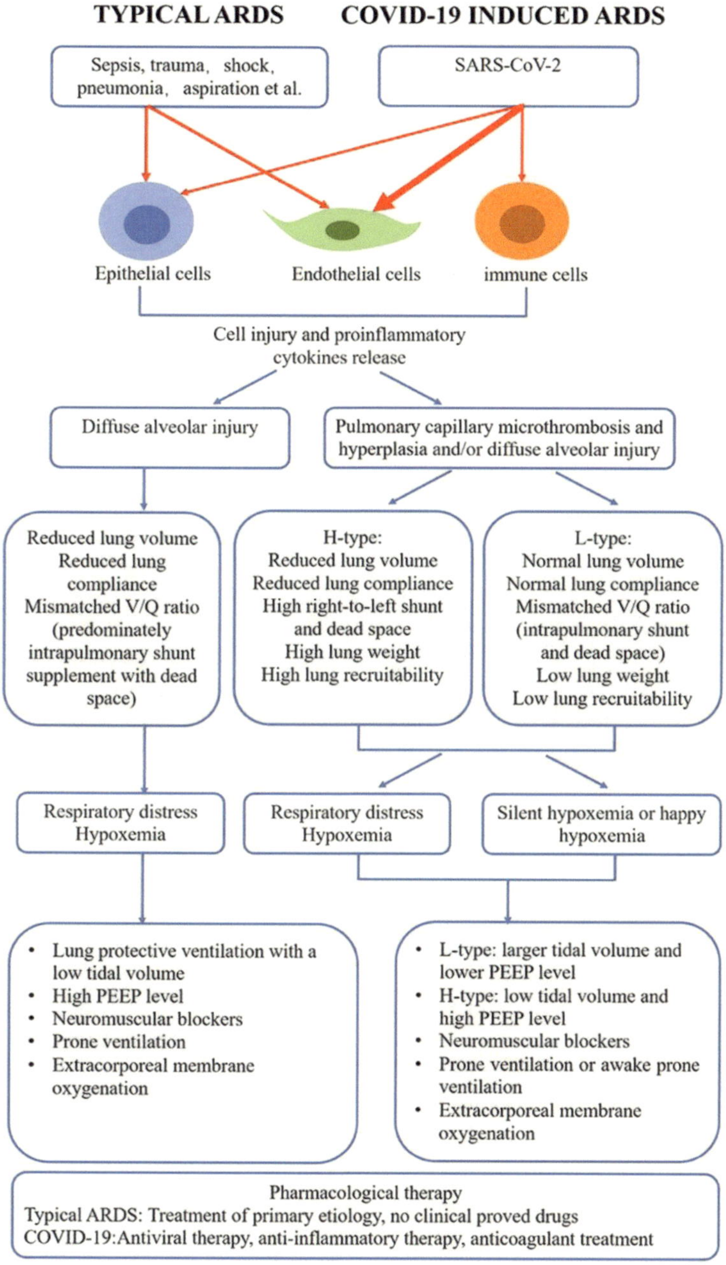

Figure 1.
Comparison of ARDS-associated and non-associated COVID-19. Source: Lu [4].

redistributing pulmonary perfusion and boosting the ratio of ventilation to perfusion. Although the venous blood mixing from right to left shunt is apparent in these individuals, about 50% of computerized tomographic scans of the two lungs have shown no notable alveolar region in these individuals [21]. The primary symptoms of H-type COVID-19 include worsening of edema of the lungs and a reduction in pulmonary gas volume, which causes an increase in stretching resistance and a reduction in pulmonary compliance, high right-to-left shunt that is brought on by the alveolar collapse in gravity-dependent areas, large lung mass, high recruit ability of the lungs. H-type and conventional severe ARDS are comparable [22]. It has been reported that 20–30% of COVID-19 patients who are hospitalized in the intensive care unit (ICU) show severe hypoxemia and lung compliance below 4 ml/cmH2O, which may indicate the existence of severe ARDS [23]. Individuals with serious hypoxemia who were hospitalized in ICU had non-invasive ventilation initiated; these patients also exhibited robust spontaneous inspiratory efforts and significant chest negative pressure. Thus, these individuals also suffer patient self-induced lung injury (P-SILI) and viral infection [24]. Many COVID-19 patients exhibited L-type in the early stages. L-type can change into H-type in the late stages of the disease due to the progression of the condition and lung damage brought on by high-stress breathing [25].

The pathophysiology of conventional ARDS and COVID-19-induced ARDS differ significantly, with the L-type of COVID-19 being the most notable variation. There are numerous explanations that could apply (**Figure 1**). Considering the etiology of ARDS, typically, shock, sepsis, transfusion, trauma, and other insults result in endothelial and epithelial damage as well as disruption of the blood-gas barrier, which increases permeability and causes the flooding of the alveolar and interstitial spaces by protein-rich fluid, resulting in low compliance, decreased lung volume, and an improper ratio of ventilation to perfusion [4]. COVID-19 pathogen is nonetheless known to be SARS-CoV-2 and the associated variations, which primarily target the endothelium *via* the ACE2 receptor with only little effects on the epithelial cell. As a result, lung compliance and volume are practically normal. Additionally, COVID-19's damaged pulmonary endothelium lost its ability to regulate lung perfusion due to hypoxic vasoconstriction, which ultimately led to the development of an intrapulmonary shunt [26, 27]. Furthermore, the COVID-19-damaged pulmonary endothelium changes from a typical anti-inflammation condition to an "active" phenotype defined by pro-adhesive qualities, inflammatory mediators production, and the development of microthrombi, which causes the amount of dead space to increase [28].

4. Hypoxemic respiratory failure in COVID-19 condition

A better understanding of the pathophysiological aspects of COVID-19 continues to ensue with the discovery of different variants of SARS-CoV-2. Viral pneumonia remains the principal complication of COVID-19 simply because it is associated with fluid retention in cells, tissues, or serous cavities of the interstices of the lungs, usually situated in the sub-pleural areas [29]. Severe hypoxemia probably occurs during the phase whereby a relative amount of lung parenchyma is involved, but the exact mechanism is not fully understood. A perturbed control of pulmonary vascular tone (vasoplegia) is, however, suggested to be the cause whereby vascular tone is not constricted despite alveolar hypoxia (**Figure 2**) [31].

The mouth, nose, or eyes are the main entry points for COVID-19 causative virus, SARS-CoV-2, into the body. The mucous membrane in the back of the throat and the

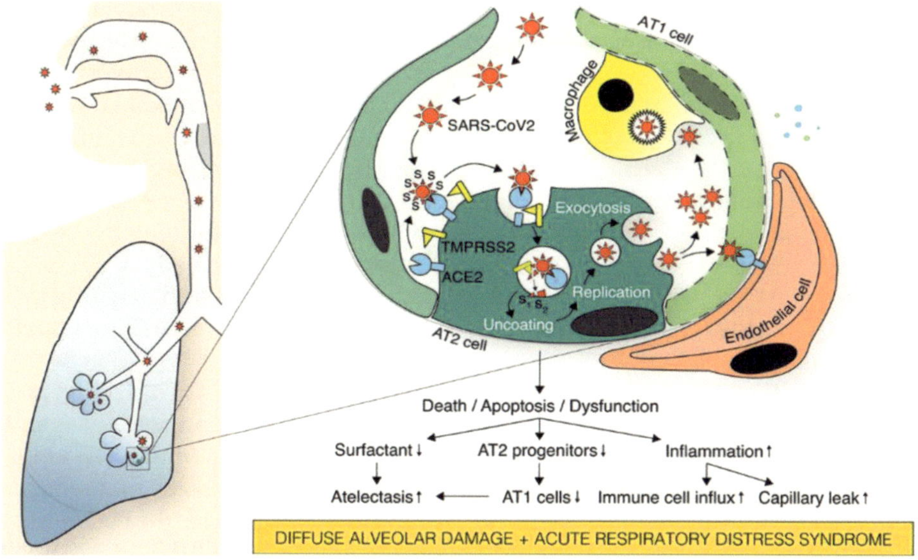

Figure 2.
Severe hypoxemia probably occurs during the phase whereby a relative amount of lung parenchyma. Source: Brosnahan [30].

rear of the nasal passages are the next places it travels. It attaches to the cells there, reproduces, and enters the lung tissue. The virus might then move on to infect further bodily tissues [32].

People who have respiratory issues can become ill from COVID-19 caused by SARS-CoV-2. The most common clinical symptom and fatality factor of COVID-19 is respiratory failure. Asymptomatic to severe respiratory failure are all possible clinical demonstrations of COVID-19. People with COVID-19-related respiratory failure may deteriorate to the point where they need invasive mechanical ventilation or may not survive [33].

Respiratory illness from mild to severe is usually experienced by most patients with virus infection who may recover without special care, while serious ailments and demand medical attention may develop in others. Serious illness is more likely to affect the elderly and people with underlying medical conditions, including cardiovascular disease, diabetes, chronic respiratory diseases, or cancer. COVID-19 has the potential to cause serious illness or kill anyone at any age [34]. Acute respiratory distress syndrome, also known as ARDS, is a serious side effect of COVID-19, and lung problems include pneumonia. There could be long-term harm to the lungs and other organs because of sepsis, another potential COVID-19 side effect. More serious respiratory diseases like bronchitis that can necessitate hospitalization may also be brought on by more recent coronavirus strains.

Lung inflammation and fluid accumulation are symptoms of pneumonia. Respiratory difficulties in certain patients can be so severe that they require medical care, oxygen therapy, and perhaps a ventilator. Pneumonia due to COVID-19 usually affects both lungs. Coughing, shortness of breath, and other symptoms appear when the fluid-filled air sacs in the lungs' ability to absorb oxygen are blocked. Despite the fact that most patients recover from COVID-19-induced pneumonia without any long-term lung damage, pneumonia can be rather severe. Lung damage may result in breathing issues even after the illness has stopped; these issues may improve over several months [34].

Bronchitis in COVID-19 conditions is associated with excessive production of sputum in the airways. The excessive sputum leads to cough and chest congestion and constricts the airways, making breathing more difficult. Even after recovery from COVID-19 infection, inflammation of the membranes lining the bronchial tubes may continue to stimulate coughing with consequential effects on the quality of life [35]. Furthermore, the alveoli are filled with fluid from the lungs'tiny blood veins as COVID-19 pneumonia advances. The resultant outcome is the development of acute respiratory distress syndrome (ARDS), which is the term for lung failure that may occur as a result of shortness of breath. In order to assist the body in circulating oxygen, many ARDS patients are unable to breathe on their own and may require ventilator support. Recovery from COVID-19 and ARDS may result in lung scarring that lasts a lifetime [36].

Severe COVID-19 infection complications include sepsis. When an infection gets into the bloodstream and circulates throughout it, causing tissue damage, sepsis starts to take hold. The collaboration between the organs breaks down in sepsis. The lungs and heart are only two examples of the many organ systems that can begin to shut down one after the other. Even in cases where sepsis is successfully treated, the patient may experience long-term lung and other organ damage [37]. In the COVID-19 condition, the immune system is actively battling the invader. This could make the body more susceptible to a superinfection—the simultaneous infection of the body with two viruses or bacteria—on top of COVID-19. Additional infections may cause more lung damage. There is a startling observation that one in four patients who get severe COVID-19 also have a superinfection, which means that their recovery will be slower [38, 39].

5. Hypoxemic respiratory failure in COVID-19

The causes of respiratory failure in COVID-19 conditions can be intrapulmonary shunting, lung perfusion regulation loss, intravascular microthrombi, impaired diffusion capacity, preservation of lung mechanics, and rapid deterioration [40].

V/Q mismatch principally causes arterial hypoxemia at the initial state of SARS-CoV-2 infection. Therefore, continuous flow of pulmonary arterial blood to the non-ventilated alveoli manifests a significant increment in P(A-a)O2 gradient, which eventually results in local interstitial edema domiciled mainly at the interface that can be termed intrapulmonary shunting [14, 30].

A proportional failure of the hypoxic pulmonary vasoconstriction mechanism or constriction of intrapulmonary arteries in alveolar hypoxia in COVID-19 condition usually causes a never-ceasing increase in the pulmonary flow of blood to nonaerated alveoli of the lung [3]. This cascade of events leads to the loss of control over lung perfusion. The resultant effect is a decreased concentration of angiotensin-converting enzyme 2 (ACE2) associated with an increased level of angiotensin II (Ang II), leading to arbitration of pulmonary vasoconstriction *via* agonist effect at the Ang II receptor, while being antagonized by Ang 1–7 [41].

Furthermore, the imbalance between fibrinolytic activity and procoagulant majorly results in intravascular microthrombi when there is severe inflammation and endothelial injury (a hallmark of COVID-19 pathogenesis). Endothelial injury can be a result affect infection of the lung capillary endothelial cells by a cytopathic virus that directly affects the expression of ACE2 [42].

It is also possible that the lung diffusion capacity is impaired due to the loss of alveolar epithelial cells from COVID-19. This results in the propagation within the alveolar cells (type II cells). In this situation, the production of many viral particles that are being released leads to an immune response that mediates the death of infected cells. This increases P(A-a)O2 gradient and arterial hypoxemia in the COVID-19 condition [12, 43].

It has also been known that there is a peak of COVID-19 challenge in patients on mechanical ventilation, signifying probably low respiratory system compliance. On the contrary, an increased airway resistance or increase in physiological and anatomical inactive ventilation usually does not occur at the onset of infection. There is also a steady breathing rate maintained at a low frequency as much as there is normality in lung compliance in patients having no underlining lung disease [44].

There can be a rapid deterioration in patients with COVID-19 that has an impact on the cortical response obtained from respiratory points. Consequently, the disease advances with a concomitant increase in dyspnea [45].

6. Clinical manifestation of respiratory failure in COVID-19

An 8- to 12-day incubation period was usually experienced by persons having COVID-19. The symptoms of COVID-19 might range from being asymptomatic and having minor symptoms to having severe ARDS. The most prevalent symptoms in patients with severe COVID-19 who needed to be admitted to the hospital were cough, fever, and dyspnea [46]. Patients with COVID-19 frequently experience extrapulmonary organ symptoms, including gastrointestinal ones like vomiting, nausea, and diarrhea, as well as taste and smell loss, headaches, bone pain, muscular aches, and other similar ones [47].

Some patients with cases of COVID-19 do not exhibit evident dyspnea while having significant hypoxemia, with oxygen saturation below 70% and partial pressure of arterial oxygen below 40 mmHg, a condition known as "silent hypoxemia" or "happy hypoxemia." The predominant partial pressure of CO_2 inhibits the reaction of the brain to hypoxia, abnormal chemoreceptor function of the carotid body caused by virus attacks, inaccurate oxygen in arterial blood at low saturations, shifts in the oxygen dissociation curve, and distinct permissiveness of low oxygen concentrations [45, 48]. Another possibility for "silent hypoxia" is a cardiorespiratory adaptation to hypoxemia. Tachycardia and increased cardiac output are the typical reactions. However, these reactions are constrained by aging, genetics, and concurrent diseases. Lactic acidosis, bradycardia, and a lower cardiac output are signs that the body is unable to make up for the reduced oxygen transfer. The latter could appear suddenly, and they are all warning signs of impending tissue damage or hypoxemia-induced mortality [49].

Because there are so many blood vessels in lung tissues, SARS-CoV-2 can directly instigate severe harm to the vascular endothelium of the lung. Variable degrees of damage are also exhibited by the airway and alveolar epithelium [50]. Endothelial cell activation potentiates inflammatory reactions and coagulation apart from participating in the adhesion, rolling, and migration of inflammatory cells. This cascade of events eventually results in coagulation activation, diffusion dysfunction, and barrier degradation [51].

Edema, infiltration of inflammatory cells, fibrinous exudation, congestion of alveolar septal vesicle, vascular thrombi, and hemorrhagic necrosis are some of the pathological symptoms of COVID-19 [52]. On postmortem, these patients had a diffuse alveolar injury (DAD) recorded in 67–100% of them, which is consistent with the usual ARDS. The COVID-19 patients did, however, exhibit specific vascular characteristics, such as microthrombosis and hyperplasia, as a result of the severe endothelium destruction. SARS-CoV-2 infection directly contributes to the development of endotheliitis in a number of organs as a result of viral participation (distinguished by the involvement of viral bodies) and the response of inflammation of the host (**Figure** 3) [4].

Studies have shown distinctive vascular features in the lungs of COVID-19 fatality patients. Capillary microthrombi of the lungs were nine times higher in COVID-19 patients than in influenza patients. It was complemented by capillary hyperplasia *via* intussusceptive angiogenesis, together with interrupted cell membranes and severe endothelial injury with an intracellular virus [53, 54]. A pulmonary embolism represented one-third of the patients' primary causes of death in an autopsy analysis of 12 consecutive COVID-19 patients. The frequency of deep thrombosis in the veins was up to 58%. These findings imply that the primary vascular alterations in COVID-19 patients, including microthrombosis of the lung capillary, damage of the epithelial cells, and hyperplasia are what distinguish them from ARDS patients and result in a distinct pathophysiological action and therapeutic feedback [55, 56]. Although the majority of patients had DAD, these data came from autopsies of people who had COVID-19-related deaths. DAD is most likely a late-stage manifestation of this illness rather than an early indicator [57].

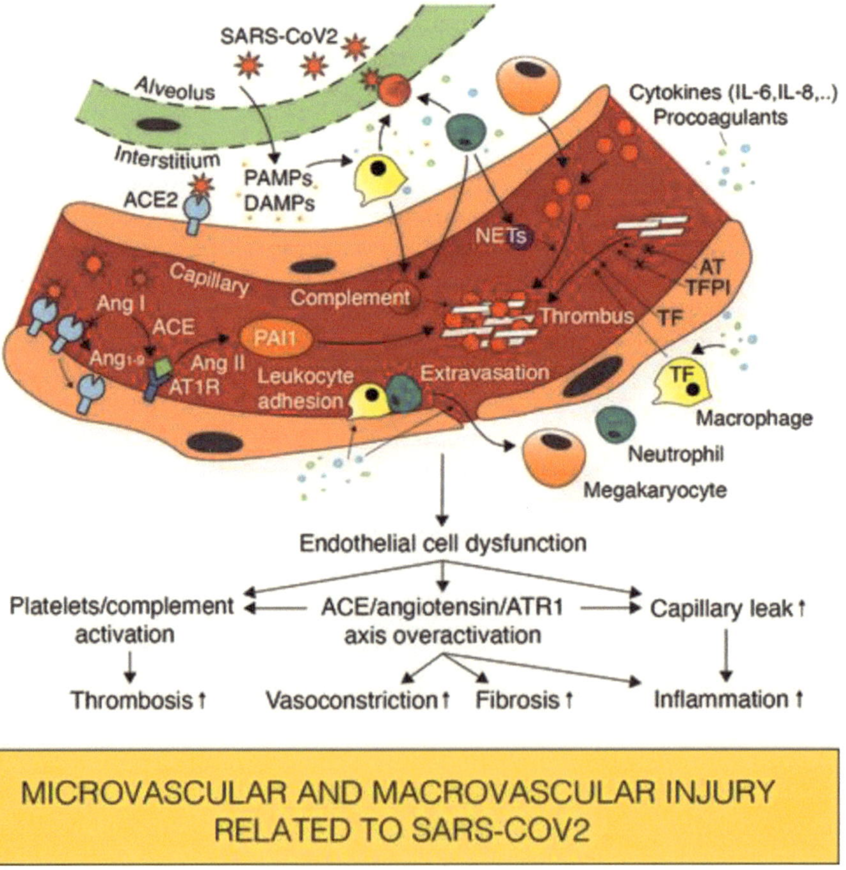

Figure 3.
Pathobiological effects of epithelial injury tiny air sacs of the lungs by acute respiratory syndrome coronavirus-2 (SARS-CoV2) infection. Source: Brosnahan [30].

7. Management of respiratory failure in COVID-19 condition

The pathology and management of hypoxemic respiratory failure in the COVID-19 condition have similarities with acute respiratory distress syndrome. Acute hypoxemic respiratory failure, often manifested as hemoglobinopathies, pulmonary edema, or vascular occlusion, is considered a grave complication of COVID-19 and requires mechanical ventilation [19].

Mechanisms (including include vascular occlusion, hemoglobinopathies, pulmonary edema, and a mismatch between ventilation and perfusion) have been proposed for the substantial hypoxemic condition in patients. However, histopathological evaluation reveals the similarity between diffuse alveolar damage or related etiologies and ARDS [58]. Also, many comparable features exist between the variable pulmonary compliance in COVID-19 and pulmonary compliance values in ARDS. As a whole, patients with COVID-19 have similar pathology to ARDS [19]. Oxygen therapy, non-invasive ventilation, and intubation are ways of managing respiratory failure in COVID-19 condition. However, there may be some factors to consider for the best management choice [59]. For instance, there is controversy about choosing between a high-flow nasal cannula (HFNC), early intubation, or non-invasive positive pressure ventilation because there are patients who may need support beyond supplemental oxygen. Protecting healthcare workers from being exposed to viral aerosols while rendering care to patients may also be another issue. Also, non-invasive positive pressure ventilation (NIPPV) usually renders ventilatory support out the requirement of the endotracheal airway, which keeps the patients awake. This management option is non-invasive, but it is not entirely benign. It has been shown that ventilation protection having minimal volumes and pressures of tide improves results in ARDS patients. By and large, management options for respiratory failure in COVID-19 range from optimized oxygenation, respiratory support availability, necessary intubation, and of course, orienting ventilatory pressure with the needs of patients [31, 60].

8. Conclusion

COVID-19, caused by SARS-CoV-2, is highly infectious that leads to the fatal coexistence of two or more related medical conditions, especially ARDS. People with respiratory issues can be vulnerable to COVID-19. Therefore, for patients with COVID-19 condition, severe hypoxemia associated with ARDS is the frontline cause of acute respiratory failure. The most prominent clinical symptom and human death factor of COVID-19 is respiratory failure. Symptomless or mild- to life-threatening respiratory failure are possible clinical manifestations of COVID-19 condition. In individuals with severe COVID-19, critical hypoxemia related to ARDS is the major causative factor of acute respiratory failure. COVID-19-associated ARDS have similarities with other causes of ARDS in relation to pathology and respiratory physiology. In this regard, patients with respiratory failure in COVID-19 conditions are usually managed as in the condition of ARDS. Since there is no clear-cut treatment for COVID-19, supportive treatment is crucial. Sound knowledge of the features of respiratory failure in COVID-19-related ARDS is crucial for accurate treatment. This review provides more scientific information on the pathophysiologic mechanisms linked with ARDS and severe COVID-19 pneumonia with emphasis on respiratory failure related to COVID-19 associated with acute hypoxemia. This will help to improve the prognosis.

Conflict of interest

The authors declare no conflict of interest.

Author details

Olalekan Bukunmi Ogunro[1*] and Oluwaseun Ruth Olasehinde[2]

1 Reproductive and Endocrinology, Toxicology, and Bioinformatics Research Laboratory, Department of Biological Sciences, KolaDaisi University, Ibadan, Oyo State, Nigeria

2 Department of Medical Biochemistry, College of Medicine and Health Science, Afe Babalola University, Ado-Ekiti, Nigeria

*Address all correspondence to: olalekanbukunmi@gmail.com

References

[1] Gyebi GA, Adegunloye AP, Ibrahim IM, Ogunyemi OM, Afolabi SO, Ogunro OB. Prevention of SARS-CoV-2 cell entry: Insight from in silico interaction of drug-like alkaloids with spike glycoprotein, human ACE2, and TMPRSS2. Journal of Biomolecular Structure and Dynamics. 2020;**40**(5):2121-2145. DOI: 10.1080/07391102.2020.1835726

[2] Gyebi GA, Ogunro OB, Adegunloye AP, Ogunyemi OM, Afolabi SO. Potential inhibitors of coronavirus 3-chymotrypsin-like protease (3CLpro): An in silico screening of alkaloids and terpenoids from African medicinal plants. Journal of Biomolecular Structure and Dynamics. 2021;**39**(9):3396-3408. DOI: 10.1080/07391102.2020.1764868

[3] Czajkowska-Malinowska M, Kania A, Kuca P, Nasiłowski J, Skoczyński S, Sokołowski R, et al. Treatment of acute respiratory failure in the course of covid-19. Practical hints from the expert panel of the assembly of intensive care and rehabilitation of the polish respiratory society. Advances. Respiratory Medicine. 2020;**88**(3):245-266

[4] Lu S, Huang X, Liu R, Lan Y, Lei Y, Zeng F, et al. Comparison of COVID-19 induced respiratory failure and typical ARDS: Similarities and differences. Frontiers in Medicine. 2022;**9**(5):1-11

[5] Oldani S, Ravaglia C, Bensai S, Bertolovic L, Ghirotti C, Puglisi S, et al. Pathophysiology of light phenotype SARS-CoV-2 interstitial pneumonia: From histopathological features to clinical presentations. Pulmonology. 2022;**28**(5):333-344. DOI: 10.1016/j.pulmoe.2021.03.003

[6] Ball L, Silva PL, Giacobbe DR, Bassetti M, Zubieta-Calleja GR, Rocco PRM, et al. Understanding the pathophysiology of typical acute respiratory distress syndrome and severe COVID-19. Expert Review of Respiratory Medicine. 2022;**16**(4): 437-446. DOI: 10.1080/17476348.2022.2057300

[7] Harless J, Ramaiah R, Bhananker SM. Pediatric airway management. International Journal of Critical Illness and Injury Science. 2014;**4**(1):65-71

[8] Wallbridge P, Steinfort D, Tay TR, Irving L, Hew M. Diagnostic chest ultrasound for acute respiratory failure. Respiratory Medicine. 2018;**141**(2):26-36. DOI: 10.1016/j.rmed.2018.06.018

[9] Piraino T. Noninvasive respiratory support in acute hypoxemic respiratory failure. Respiratory Care. 2019;**64**(6):638-646

[10] Kempker JA, Abril MK, Chen Y, Kramer MR, Waller LA, Martin GS. The epidemiology of respiratory failure in the United States 2002-2017: A serial cross-sectional study. Critical Care Explorations. 2020;**2**(6):e0128. DOI: 10.1097/CCE.0000000000000128

[11] Rochwerg B, Brochard L, Elliott MW, Hess D, Hill NS, Nava S, et al. Official ERS/ATS clinical practice guidelines: Noninvasive ventilation for acute respiratory failure. European Respiratory Journal. 2017;**50**(4):1-20. DOI: 10.1183/13993003.02426-2016

[12] Clementi N, Ghosh S, De Santis M, Castelli M, Criscuolo E, Zanoni I, et al. Viral respiratory pathogens and lung injury. Clinical Microbiology Reviews. 2021;**34**(3):e00103-e00120. DOI: 10.1128/CMR.00103-20

[13] Laghi F, Tobin MJ. Disorders of the respiratory muscles. American Journal of Respiratory and Critical Care Medicine. 2003;**168**(1):10-48

[14] Sarkar M, Niranjan N, Banyal PK. Mechanisms of hypoxemia. Lung India. 2017;**34**(1):47-60

[15] Kershaw CD, Guidot DM. Alcoholic lung disease. Alcohol Research and Health. 2008;**31**(1):66-75

[16] Gottlieb J, Capetian P, Hamsen U, Janssens U, Karagiannidis C, Kluge S, et al. German S3 guideline: Oxygen therapy in the acute care of adult patients. Respiration. 2022;**101**(2):214-252

[17] Li C, He Q, Qian H, Liu J. Overview of the pathogenesis of COVID-19 (Review). Experimental and Therapeutic Medicine. 2021;**22**(3):1-10

[18] Pfortmueller CA, Spinetti T, Urman RD, Luedi MM, Schefold JC. COVID-19-associated acute respiratory distress syndrome (CARDS): Current knowledge on pathophysiology and ICU treatment - a narrative review. Best Practice & Research Clinical Anaesthesiology. 2021;**35**(3):351-368. DOI: 10.1016/j.bpa.2020.12.011

[19] Swenson KE, Ruoss SJ, Swenson ER. The pathophysiology and dangers of silent hypoxemia in COVID-19 lung injury. Annals of the American Thoracic Society. 2021;**18**(7):1098-1105

[20] Gattinoni L, Chiumello D, Rossi S. COVID-19 pneumonia: ARDS or not? Critical Care. 2020;**24**(1):1-3

[21] Marini JJ, Hotchkiss JR, Broccard AF. Bench-to-bedside review: Microvascular and airspace linkage in ventilator-induced lung injury. Clinical Review & Education. 2020;**323**(22):2329-2330

[22] Karbing DS, Panigada M, Bottino N, Spinelli E, Protti A, Rees SE, et al. Changes in shunt, ventilation/perfusion mismatch, and lung aeration with PEEP in patients with ARDS: A prospective single-arm interventional study. Critical Care. 2020;**24**(1):1-13

[23] Krynytska I, Marushchak M, Birchenko I, Dovgalyuk A, Tokarskyy O. COVID-19-associated acute respiratory distress syndrome versus classical acute respiratory distress syndrome (a narrative review). Iranian Journal of Microbiology. 2021;**13**(6):737-747

[24] Fernando SM, Ferreyro BL, Urner M, Munshi L, Fan E. Diagnosis and management of acute respiratory distress syndrome. CMAJ. 2021;**193**(21):E761-E768

[25] Sharma G, Goodwin J. Effect of aging on respiratory system physiology and immunology. Clinical interventions in Aging. 2006;**1**(3):253-260

[26] Barbosa LC, Gonçalves TL, de Araujo LP, de Rosario LV, Ferrer VP. Endothelial cells and SARS-CoV-2: An intimate relationship. Vascular Pharmacology. 2021;**137**(1):106829. DOI: 10.1016/j.vph.2021.106829

[27] Kumar A, Singh R, Kaur J, Pandey S, Sharma V, Thakur L, et al. Wuhan to world: The COVID-19 pandemic. Frontiers in Cellular and Infection Microbiology. 2021;**11**(3):1-21

[28] Smadja DM, Mentzer SJ, Fontenay M, Laffan MA, Ackermann M, Helms J, et al. COVID-19 Is a Systemic Vascular Hemopathy: Insight for Mechanistic and Clinical Aspects. Vol. 24. Netherlands: Springer; 2021. pp. 755-788. DOI: 10.1007/s10456-021-09805-6

[29] Alipoor SD, Jamaati H, Tabarsi P, Mortaz E. Immunopathogenesis of

pneumonia in covid-19. Tanaffos. 2020;**19**(2):79-82

[30] Brosnahan SB, Jonkman AH, Kugler MC, Munger JS, Kaufman DA. COVID-19 and respiratory system disorders: Current knowledge, future clinical and translational research questions. Arteriosclerosis, Thrombosis, and Vascular Biology. 2020;**40**(11):2586-2597

[31] Raoof S, Nava S, Carpati C, Hill NS. High-flow, noninvasive ventilation and awake (nonintubation) Proning in patients with coronavirus disease 2019 with respiratory failure. Chest. 2020;**158**(5):1992-2002. DOI: 10.1016/j.chest.2020.07.013

[32] Wiersinga WJ, Rhodes A, Cheng AC, Peacock SJ, Prescott HC. Pathophysiology, transmission, diagnosis, and treatment of coronavirus disease 2019 (COVID-19): A review. JAMA - Journal of the American Medical Association. 2020;**324**(8):782-793

[33] Lotfi M, Hamblin MR, Rezaei N. COVID-19: Transmission, prevention, and potential therapeutic opportunities. Clinica Chimica Acta. 2020;**508**(4):254-266

[34] Attaway AH, Scheraga RG, Bhimraj A, Biehl M, Hatipoğ LU. Severe covid-19 pneumonia: Pathogenesis and clinical management. The. BMJ. 2021;**372**:n436. DOI: 10.1136/bmj.n436

[35] Goyal D, Inada-Kim M, Mansab F, Iqbal A, McKinstry B, Naasan AP, et al. Improving the early identification of COVID-19 pneumonia: A narrative review. BMJ Open Respiratory Research. 2021;**8**(1):1-9

[36] Gibson PG, Qin L, Puah SH. COVID-19 acute respiratory distress syndrome (ARDS): Clinical features and differences from typical pre-COVID-19 ARDS. Medical Journal of Australia. 2020;**213**(2):54-56.e1

[37] Olwal CO, Nganyewo NN, Tapela K, Djomkam Zune AL, Owoicho O, Bediako Y, et al. Parallels in sepsis and COVID-19 conditions: Implications for managing severe COVID-19. Frontiers in Immunology. 2021;**12**(2):1-6

[38] Hoque MN, Akter S, Dilruba I, Islam MR. Microbial co-infections in COVID-19: Associated microbiota and underlying mechanisms of pathogenesis. Microbial Pathogenesis. 2021;**156**:104941. DOI: 10.1016/j.micpath.2021.104941

[39] Schultze JL, Aschenbrenner AC. COVID-19 and the human innate immune system. Cell. 2021;**184**(7):1671-1692. DOI: 10.1016/j.cell.2021.02.029

[40] Yuan S, Jiang SC, Zhang ZW, Fu YF, Hu J, Li ZL. The role of alveolar edema in covid-19. Cell. 2021;**10**(8):1-15

[41] Ni W, Yang X, Yang D, Bao J, Li R, Xiao Y, et al. Role of angiotensin-converting enzyme 2 (ACE2) in COVID-19. Critical Care. 2020;**24**(1):1-10

[42] Prasad M, Leon M, Lerman LO, Lerman A. Viral endothelial dysfunction: A unifying mechanism for COVID-19. Mayo Clinic Proceedings 2021;9(12):3099-3108. A

[43] Fuschillo S, Ambrosino P, Motta A, Maniscalco M. COVID-19 and diffusing capacity of the lungs for carbon monoxide: A clinical biomarker in care settings. Biomarkers in Medicine. 2021;**15**(8):2-4

[44] Haudebourg AF, Perier F, Tuffet S, De Prost N, Razazi K, Dessap AM, et al. Respiratory mechanics of COVID-19- versus non-COVID-19-associated acute

respiratory distress syndrome. American Journal of Respiratory and Critical Care Medicine. 2020;**202**(2):287-290

[45] Dhont S, Derom E, Van Braeckel E, Depuydt P, Lambrecht BN. Conceptions of the pathophysiology of happy hypoxemia in COVID-19. Respiratory Research. 2021;**22**(1):1-9

[46] Lauer SA, Grantz KH, Bi Q, Jones FK, Zheng Q, Meredith HR, et al. The incubation period of coronavirus disease 2019 (CoVID-19) from publicly reported confirmed cases: Estimation and application. Annals of Internal Medicine. 2020;**172**(9):577-582

[47] Sarkesh A, Sorkhabi AD, Sheykhsaran E, Alinezhad F, Mohammadzadeh N, Hemmat N, et al. Extrapulmonary clinical manifestations in COVID-19 patients. American Journal of Tropical Medicine and Hygiene. 2020;**103**(5):1783-1796

[48] Bickler PE, Feiner JR, Lipnick MS, McKleroy W. "Silent" presentation of hypoxemia and cardiorespiratory compensation in COVID-19. Anesthesiology. 2021;**134**(2):262-269. DOI: 10.1097/ALN.0000000000003578

[49] Stawicki S, Jeanmonod R, Miller A, Paladino L, Gaieski D, Yaffee A, et al. The 2019-2020 novel coronavirus (severe acute respiratory syndrome coronavirus 2) pandemic: A joint american college of academic international medicine-world academic council of emergency medicine multidisciplinary COVID-19 working group consensus paper. Journal of Global Infectious Diseases. 2020;**12**(2):47-93

[50] Jin Y, Ji W, Yang H, Chen S, Zhang W, Duan G. Endothelial activation and dysfunction in COVID-19: From basic mechanisms to potential therapeutic approaches. Signal Transduction and Targeted Therapy. 2020;**5**(1):1-13. DOI: 10.1038/s41392-020-00454-7

[51] Stenmark KR, Frid MG, Gerasimovskaya E, Zhang H, McCarthy MK, Thurman JM, et al. Mechanisms of SARS-CoV-2-induced lung vascular disease: potential role of complement. Pulmonary Circulation. 2021;**11**(2):1-14. DOI: 10.1177/20458940211015799

[52] Mondello C, Roccuzzo S, Malfa O, Sapienza D, Gualniera P, Ventura Spagnolo E, et al. Pathological findings in COVID-19 as a tool to define SARS-CoV-2 pathogenesis. A systematic review. Frontiers in Pharmacology. 2021;**12(4)12**:614586. DOI: 10.3389/fphar.2021.614586

[53] Bösmüller H, Matter M, Fend F, Tzankov A. The pulmonary pathology of COVID-19. Virchows Archives. 2021;**478**(1):137-150

[54] Ackermann M, Verleden SE, Kuehnel M, Haverich A, Welte T, Laenger F, et al. Pulmonary vascular Endothelialitis, thrombosis, and angiogenesis in Covid-19. New England Journal of Medicine. 2020;**383**(2):120-128

[55] Deshpande C. Thromboembolic findings in COVID-19 autopsies: Pulmonary thrombosis or embolism? Annals of Internal Medicine. 2020;**173**(5):394-395

[56] Wichmann D, Sperhake JP, Lütgehetmann M, Steurer S, Edler C, Heinemann A, et al. Autopsy findings and venous thromboembolism in patients with COVID-19: A prospective cohort study. Annals of Internal Medicine. 2020;**173**(4):268-277

[57] Elsoukkary SS, Mostyka M, Dillard A, Berman DR, Ma LX, Chadburn A, et al. Autopsy findings in 32 patients with COVID-19: A single-institution experience. Pathobiology. 2021;**88**(1):56-68

[58] Wilcox SR. Management of respiratory failure due to covid-19. The BMJ. 2020;**369**(5):2-3. DOI: 10.1136/bmj.m1786

[59] Bonnesen B, Jensen JUS, Jeschke KN, Mathioudakis AG, Corlateanu A, Hansen EF, et al. Management of covid-19-associated acute respiratory failure with alternatives to invasive mechanical ventilation: High-flow oxygen, continuous positive airway pressure, and noninvasive ventilation. Diagnostics. 2021;**11**(12):1-12

[60] Mina B, Newton A, Hadda V. Noninvasive ventilation in treatment of respiratory failure-related COVID-19 infection: Review of the literature. Canadian Respiratory Journal. 2022;**9914081**(8):1-8. DOI: 10.1155/2022/9914081

Section 4

Respiratory Failure in Specialized Conditions

Chapter 5

Pulmonary Issues in Chronic Liver Disease

Vijay Kant Pandey, Aaditya Anil Prabhudesai and Subhash Gupta

Abstract

Pulmonary complications are important cause for high incidence of mortality in chronic liver disease patients admitted to the intensive care unit. Up to 50–70% of patients report shortness of breath, reflecting the high prevalence of respiratory failure, defined as an arterial pressure of oxygen (PaO_2) of less than 60 mm Hg. The causes of respiratory failure are multifactorial in chronic liver disease. Although much attention is given to the pathologies of pulmonary microcirculation (i.e., portopulmonary hypertension and hepatopulmonary syndrome), these specific conditions are found in <20% of cirrhotic patients. The impact of liver disease on respiratory function extends far beyond these two specific conditions and include micro-aspirations associated with hepatic encephalopathy, fluid overload, hepatic hydrothorax, and basal atelectasis and restriction due to large ascites. The impact of altered bile-acid composition induces a shift in the gut microbiome and this may shed a new light on the molecular basis for the 'gut–liver–lung axis' as the driver for multiple organ failure. This chapter focuses on current evidence surrounding the prevalence, management, and complications from various etiologies of respiratory insufficiency in end-stage liver disease patients.

Keywords: chronic liver disease (CLD), portal hypertension, pulmonary hypertension, portopulmonary hypertension, hepatopulmonary syndrome, hepatic hydrothorax

1. Introduction

Pulmonary disorder in liver disease can broadly be classified into the following 3 groups:

1. Pulmonary disorders which are direct sequelae of liver disease and portal hypertension (hepatopulmonary syndrome (HPS), portopulmonary hypertension (POPH), and hepatic hydrothorax (HH)

2. Coexisting common respiratory disease (i.e., asthma, chronic obstructive pulmonary disease (COPD), interstitial lung disease) along with pulmonary disease specific to liver disease

3. Disorders that affect both liver and lungs (Alpha-1 antitrypsin deficiency, cystic fibrosis, sarcoidosis, hereditary hemorrhagic telangiectasia)

Chronic liver disease (CLD) and portal hypertension are associated with an imbalance between vasoconstrictors and vasodilators leading to hyperdynamic circulation from splanchnic and systemic vasodilatation. This continued exposure to vasoactive and proliferative mediators leads to remodelling processes in the pulmonary vascular bed, either in the form of diffuse telangiectasia (in HPS) or hyperplastic lesions in terminal pulmonary arterioles (in POPH) [1]. Effect of these pulmonary vascular and parenchymal abnormalities is further augmented by mechanical restriction due to ascites. The spectrum of presentation of these respiratory insufficiencies is varied, with differences in symptoms, signs, pulmonary function tests, ultrasound findings, and gas exchange abnormalities.

Although HPS and POPH are widely discussed in the literature, finding an isolated pulmonary abnormality in end-stage liver disease is rare in real clinical circumstances. There can be multiple diseases (pleural effusion and HPS, or COPD and POPH) coexisting in the same patient. Identifying different contributors, quantifying their severity, and their impact on overall clinical picture is important for patients' symptomatic treatment, optimization before transplantation, and perioperative management.

A comprehensive understanding of potential respiratory pathophysiology that may complicate liver disease and liver transplantation (LT) is essential with the aim of inclusive management. Disorders that affect both the liver and lungs are beyond the scope of this book chapter. This chapter will deal with chronic liver disease's direct and indirect effects leading to respiratory insufficiency.

2. Hepatopulmonary syndrome

HPS is an oxygenation defect occurring in patients with liver disease and/or portal hypertension resulting from intrapulmonary vascular dilatations (IPVDs). HPS may also manifest in acute liver failure, ischemic or viral hepatitis, and portal vein thrombosis. The prevalence of HPS is around 5–30%, while isolated vasodilatation can be found in up to 60% cirrhotic without evidence of arterial hypoxemia [2]. HPS is a progressive disease, and gradual deterioration occurs in 87% of cases with a monthly decline in PaO_2 of 1.1 ± 1.4 mm Hg [3]. Patients with HPS are frequently asymptomatic, resulting in under-recognition of the disease and a delay in diagnosis. This delay in diagnosis and LT is associated with increased mortality [2].

2.1 Suspecting the possibility of HPS

The typical symptom of HPS is dyspnoea on exertion (DOE) and in severe cases Dyspnoea at rest. However, DOE is nonspecific in the case of cirrhosis, and HPS patients may be asymptomatic at mild to moderate severity. This indicates that we should actively screen the patients with cirrhosis for HPS. Clinical signs may include digital clubbing, cyanosis, and diffuse telangiectasias. Although classically described in HPS, **platypnea** (dyspnoea worsening when moving from supine to upright position) and **orthodeoxia** (>5% or >4 mm Hg decrease in SPO_2 or PaO_2, respectively, after changing from supine to upright position) is observed in only in 18–20% of patients with HPS [4]. The coexistence of other pulmonary diseases, such as including COPD, asthma, and interstitial lung disease, should be investigated, as they may exacerbate clinical symptoms and gas exchange abnormalities.

2.2 Screening

Pulse oximetry is easy to use, readily available and is a cost-effective tool to identify hypoxemia. Oxygen saturation < 96% identifies all patients with hypoxemia (PaO_2 < 70 mm Hg) at sea level [5]. In cirrhotic children hyperaemic arterialized capillary blood gas determination found better screening tool than pulse oximetry [6]. A recent study has found that pulse oximetry is an insensitive screening test for severe HPS in LT candidates and showed that a SaO_2 of 94% provides poor sensitivity (22.1%) and specificity (89.8%) to detect severe HPS [7]. However, pulse oximetry seems to be a widely accepted tool to exclude the diagnosis of HPS. To detect all patients with HPS, ABG analysis should be done if oxygen saturation <96%.

2.3 Diagnostic criteria

The hallmark of HPS is intrapulmonary vascular dilatations (IPVDs) which leads to oxygenation defect in the setting of advanced liver disease, portal hypertension, or congenital portosystemic shunts. Abnormal oxygenation is defined by an elevated resting alveolar-arterial oxygen gradient [P(A-a) $O_2 \geq 15$ mm Hg or ≥20 mm Hg if age >64 years] while breathing room air in the sitting position, in the absence of other than mild pulmonary function test abnormalities (**Table 1**) [1, 2]. IVPDs can be demonstrated by contrast-enhanced transthoracic echocardiography (CE-TTE) or Technetium-99 m (Tc99m) labelled macro-aggregated albumin (MAA) lung perfusion scan [8]. **Table 1** enumerates the diagnostic criteria for HPS.

The severity of HPS is determined by the degree of hypoxemia on arterial blood gas. Based on the European respiratory society (ERS) Task Force, severity is graded as mild ($PaO_2 \geq 80$ mm Hg), moderate (PaO_2 = 60–79 mm Hg), severe (PaO_2 = 50–59 mm Hg), and very severe (PaO_2 < 50 mm Hg) [8]. So PaO2 is not essential to diagnose HPS, it is required to classify for severity of HPS.

Despite well-defined criteria for its diagnosis, HPS is often inaccurately diagnosed because of the lack of use of standard diagnostic criteria, or attempt to diagnose and classify during acute illness, and sometimes from diagnostic confusion with POPH and

	Diagnostic criteria	Investigations
1	Abnormal oxygenation defined by elevated alveolar-arterial oxygen gradient (≥15 mm Hg or ≥20 mm Hg if age >64 years), in the **absence of other than mild pulmonary function test abnormalities**[a]	Arterial blood gas analysis while patient breathing room air, in sitting position at rest
2	Presence of liver disease and or portal hypertension/ portosystemic shunts	Clinical diagnosis (ascites, gastroesophageal varices, splenomegaly) or portal pressure
3	Demonstration of Intrapulmonary vasodilatations	Positive CE-TTE or >6% brain uptake on Tc99m MAA lung perfusion scan

[a]Other than mild pulmonary function test abnormalities: A forced vital capacity <70% of predicted for restrictive ventilatory defect. The obstructive ventilatory defect can be defined by a forced expiratory volume in 1 second/forced vital capacity ratio <0.70 together with forced expiratory volume in 1 second percent predicted <80%. CE-TTE (contrast-enhanced transthoracic echocardiography).

Table 1.
Diagnostic criteria for HPS.

other associated respiratory diseases. Therefore, it is important that diagnostic criteria be carefully applied whilst simultaneously demonstrating the absence or only presence of mild form of coexisting pulmonary disease [9].

The response to 100% inspired oxygen is much better in patients with HPS alone as compared to HPS with an additional pulmonary disease and it should be used whenever in doubt [9]. The response to 100% oxygen may also have prognostic importance as it demonstrates significant scope of improvement in oxygenation.

2.4 HPS vascular patterns

On the basis of pulmonary angiographic findings, HPS can be divided into Type I and II (**Table 2** describe pulmonary angiographic patterns of HPS). On the basis of, response to 100% inspired oxygen ($PaO_2 < 300$ mm Hg) and presence of discrete abnormalities on high-resolution chest computed tomography, subgroup of patients can be identified who should proceed to get pulmonary angiography [10]. Rarely coil embolization can be successfully used to improve hypoxemia in type I (diffuse) and type II (discrete) HPS [11].

2.5 Demonstration of IPVDs

IPVDs can be demonstrated non-invasively by saline contrast enhanced transthoracic echocardiography or invasively by 99mTc labelled macro-aggregated albumin (MAA) lung perfusion scan.

2.5.1 Contrast-enhanced transthoracic echocardiography (CE-TTE)

The normal diameter of pulmonary capillaries is less than 8 to 15 μm [12]. The size of microbubbles created by saline agitation is more than 10 μm in diameter, which due to greater size, does not cross through the normal pulmonary capillary vasculature after intravenous injection. The delayed appearance of these microbubbles in the left heart after 3 or more cardiac cycles after visualization in the right heart demonstrates IPVDs. CE-TTE can differentiate between IPVDs and intracardiac shunts (i.e., due to persistent foramen ovale or atrial septal defect). In intracardiac shunts microbubbles appear early in the left heart (i.e., within 1–2 cardiac cycles) [13]. It is minimally invasive, radially available and highly sensitive examination and is gold standard for demonstrating IPVDs. CE-TTE also has some limitations. For example, positive detection rate is 40%, in patients who have normal arterial blood gas content. Therefore, demonstrating IPVDs, using CE-TTE alone is not sufficient for the diagnosis of HPS [9].

	Angiographic finding	Symptoms	Response to 100% Oxygen
Type 1 minimal	Finely diffuse, spidery vascular abnormality	Hypoxemia	Excellent
Type 1 advanced (evolves from type 1 minimal	Diffuse spongy or blotchy appearance	Severe hypoxemia	Limited response
Type 2	Discrete, direct arteriovenous communications	Severe hypoxemia	Extremely poor response

Table 2.
Pulmonary angiographic patterns of HPS [10].

2.5.2 Nuclear/invasive testing

Another method to demonstrate IPVDs is lung perfusion scanning (peripheral venous injection of 20 μm 99mTechnetium labelled macro-aggregated albumin [MAA] with brain uptake >6%). Although this can quantify the IPVDs, it does not differentiate between intracardiac and intrapulmonary shunting and has lower sensitivity as compared to CE-TTE for the detection of mild or moderate HPS in adults. In children, MAA lung perfusion scans may have favourable sensitivity for detecting mild degrees of IPVD relative to CE-TTE. In HPS patients with coexisting respiratory problems abnormal brain uptake of 99mTcMAA after lung perfusion (uptake >6%) helps to distinguish and quantify the degree of hypoxemia caused by IPVDs versus hypoxemia due to nonvascular lung parenchymal abnormalities [13]. Although sensitivity of 99mTc-MAA is lower than that of CE-TTE, its specificity is higher for the diagnosis of HPS [9]. Whole-body uptake (>42.5%) of 99mTc-MAA was found superior to simple brain uptake (>5.8%) for demonstrating IPVDs [14].

2.6 Pathogenesis

The oxygenation defect in HPS has been ascribed to 3 mechanisms resulting from alterations in the alveolar microcirculation

i. Diffusion limitation

ii. Presence of direct arteriovenous communications

iii. Ventilation perfusion (V/Q) mismatch

Diffusion limitation occurs because oxygen needs to travels a more distance to bind hemoglobin due to vascular dilation. Direct arteriovenous communications bypass the alveolar microcirculation, resulting in the direct mixing of venous and arterial blood. V/Q mismatch is consequence of increased pulmonary blood flow due to microvascular alterations as compared to unchanged ventilation [15].

Work in the common bile duct model (CBDL) has identified underlying pathophysiologic triggers for 3 mechanisms that contribute to the development of hypoxemia in the HPS [16]:

1. Relaxation of blood vessels leading to vasodilation,

2. Angiogenesis leads to shunt formation, and

3. Alveolar dysfunction.

Endothelin-1 (ET-1) induced pulmonary vascular relaxation: Circulating ET-1 levels which increases in cirrhosis, has differential action on the sinusoidal and pulmonary vasculature. Although it acts as a potent vasoconstrictor for sinusoidal vasculature and increases sinusoidal and presinusoidal pressure, it causes nitric oxide (NO) mediated pulmonary vasodilatation [15].

Bacterial translocation, endotoxemia, and pulmonary inflammation: Due to portosystemic shunts bacterial translocation products and endotoxins reach the pulmonary circulation, where they induce the local release of chemotactic factors, which then recruit immune cells. Pulmonary vascular monocytes in experimental HPS models have been found to increase production of inducible nitric oxide synthase and heme-oxygenase 1, leading to NO-mediated vasodilation and, increased production of the vasodilator carbon monoxide [15].

Angiogenesis and intrapulmonary shunt formation and Alveolar dysfunction: Increased pulmonary expression of proangiogenic factors occurs in HPS, which leads to angiogenesis and formation of intrapulmonary shunts [15].

2.7 HPS and liver transplantation

Liver transplantation (LT) is only definitive therapeutic option for HPS. Previously very severe hypoxemia (PaO_2 < 50 mm Hg) due to HPS was considered an absolute contraindication for LT [17]. However, further evidence showed that LT improves IPVDs, oxygenation, and even leads to complete resolution of HPS. HPS with PaO_2 < 60 mm Hg is eligible for MELD exception points to facilitate early transplant [18].

Hypoxemia associated with HPS is progressive and with worsening severity the risk of pre- and post-LT mortality increase [19]. In HPS patients with similar baseline PaO_2, brain uptake of 99mTcMAA and liver dysfunction, 5-year survival associated with LT found to be 76% versus 23% without LT [17]. Improvement in PaO_2 can be seen in all patients after LT by 12 months and subsequent normalization of the 99mTcMAA brain scan [17]. Once MELD exception points were implemented, both survival rates and post-transplant oxygenation improved in adults whereas only post-transplant oxygenation improved in children after LT [13].

A multivariate analysis of United Network for Organ Sharing (UNOS) data regarding MELD exception points granted to HPS patients found no association between waitlist mortality and severe hypoxemia, but a pre-LT PaO_2 < 45 mm Hg was associated with increased post-LT mortality [20]. In analysis of 1152 HPS patients listed for liver transplantation, there was high likelihood of getting transplanted if patient PaO2 < 45 mm Hg. After LT, patients with a PaO_2 < 45 mm Hg had lower long-term survival, however this difference became significant only after 2.6 years. The median survival was 11.5 years in this subgroup. This suggests that in patients with very severe HPS transplant may not provide long term survival benefit but they do benefit from LT [21].

In experienced centres, HPS patients with very severe hypoxemia ($PaO_2 \leq 50$ mm Hg) and oxygen dependence showed an overall survival of 86%, comparable to non-HPS patients undergoing LT. PaO_2 improved in all patients from a mean of 65.1 to 90.9 mm Hg, and all patients dependent on ambulatory oxygen were able to discontinue oxygen therapy [3].

2.8 Salient management points

Perioperative and intensive care management concerns in HPS patients who are going for LT are mainly related to hypoxemia. Following are some general guidelines that can be used during managing HPS patients:

i. Restrictive fluid therapy should be done to avoid fluid overload and pulmonary congestion.

ii. The choice of volatile anesthetic agents does not affect oxygenation

iii. Continuous monitoring of mixed venous oxygen saturation (SvO_2) should be carried out. If the mixed venous saturation falls below 65% on hepatic vascular exclusion, veno-venous bypass may be beneficial [22].

iv. Low tidal lung protective ventilation in a supine position should be employed

v. Early extubation should be done to prevent ventilator-associated pneumonia

vi. O_2 saturation should be maintained ≥85% with supplemental oxygen

vii. Due to chronic hypoxia, HPS patients develop an increase in hemoglobin, so their hemoglobin targets should be kept higher.

viii. Inhaled pulmonary vasodilators (nitric oxide) can be used to improve post-LT oxygenation

ix. ECMO can be used as a bridge to LT

x. Supplemental oxygen should be discontinued when O_2 saturation remains greater than 88% (rest, exercise, and sleep)

xi. High frequency nasal cannula and non-invasive ventilation should also be utilized to improve oxygenation

2.9 Severe post-transplant hypoxemia

Severe post-transplant hypoxemia is defined as need of 100% oxygen to maintain a saturation of ≥85% and this hypoxemia is out of proportion to any concurrent lung process. It occurs in 6–21% of patients with HPS after liver transplantation. It is associated with a peri-transplant mortality rate of 45% in patients with pretransplant $PaO_2 < 70$ mm Hg. Due to impaired hypoxic vasoconstriction in the dilated pulmonary vasculature and disproportionately increased vasoconstriction in normal pulmonary vasculature there is increased blood flow through the dilated vessels which results in enhanced worsening of V/Q mismatch is proposed mechanism for severe post-transplant hypoxemia. Trendelenburg position, pulmonary vasodilators, inhaled nitric oxide, intravenous methylene blue, and beta-blockers can be used to maintain oxygenation [23]. Non-invasive ventilation and high frequency nasal cannula can also be used to maintain oxygenation. Extracorporeal membrane oxygenation (ECMO) showed good outcomes in patients with HPS either as a bridge to LT or to aid recovery after LT with a median ECMO duration of 13 days and survival of 82.4%. ECMO is found to improve outcome in severe HPS as compared to other indications in LT [24].

3. Pulmonary hypertension (PH) and portopulmonary hypertension (PoPH)

3.1 Definition

Pulmonary arterial hypertension (PAH) which is secondary to portal hypertension is termed portopulmonary hypertension (PoPH). The elevation of mean pulmonary artery pressures (mPAP) is because of an increase in pulmonary vascular resistance

(PVR) with normal pulmonary artery wedge pressure (PAWP). PoPH hemodynamic diagnostic criteria are derived from Right heart catheterization (RHC) enumerated in **Table 3**. To diagnose PoPH all hemodynamic criteria should be met.

3.2 Severity of PoPH

Based on the mean values of pulmonary artery pressure on RHC, PoPH is classified as mild ($25 \leq$ mPAP < 35 mm Hg), moderate ($35 \leq$ mPAP < 45 mm Hg), and severe (MPAP ≥ 45 mm Hg). In contrast to HPS, there is no association between the severity of PoPH with the disease state of CLD [13].

3.3 New developments in pulmonary hypertension

Since 1st World Symposium on Pulmonary Hypertension (WSPH) in 1973, PH has been defined as mPAP $\geqslant 25$ mm Hg measured by RHC [25]. It was recognized that this upper limit of normal mPAP of 25 mm Hg was empirical and arbitrarily defined [26]. This definition remained unchanged and was adapted by liver transplant societies [13].

Recently, 6th World Symposium on Pulmonary Hypertension (WSPH) has reconsidered the hemodynamic definition of PH and decreased the threshold for PH (mPAP$\geq$20 mm Hg) but kept PVR $>$ 3 WU for precapillary PH [25]. This reconsideration was based upon a systemic review finding that mPAP at rest is 14.0 ± 3.3 mm Hg [27]. Two standard deviations of this, would suggest mPAP ≥ 20 mm Hg as upper limit of normal. This new cut-off (mPAP ≥ 20 mm Hg) to define PH is evidence based [25].

The new definitions of PH have been endorsed and expanded in guidelines proposed by the European Respiratory Society/European Society of Cardiology, including a revised cut-off mPAP but they also reduced the PVR cut off to >2 WU [28]. (New definition of PH shown in **Figure 1**.) These hemodynamic definitions are currently not adapted by liver transplant societies. Till this update is incorporated into liver transplantation assessment, we should use the definition adapted by International liver transplant society (ILTS) and shown in **Table 3**. However hemodynamic characterization into precapillary, isolated postcapillary, and combined post-precapillary PH can be done in CLD patients using cut-off given in **Table 3**.

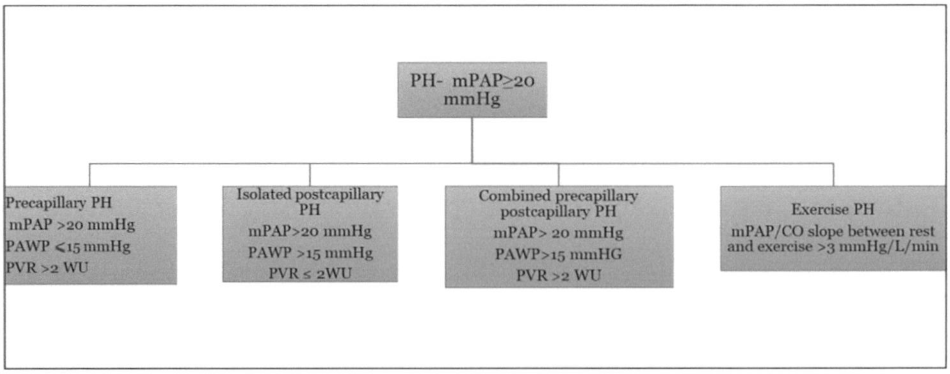

Figure 1.
New Hemodynamic definitions of pulmonary hypertension.

Portal hypertension (clinical diagnosis by gastroesophageal varices, splenomegaly, ascites) or portal pressure measurement	
mPAP >25 mm Hg	Hemodynamic parameters on Right heart catheterization with patient supine and at rest
PVR > 3 wood units (240 dynes/s per cm^{-5})	
PAWP < 15 mm Hg	

Table 3.
Diagnostic criteria for portopulmonary hypertension.

3.4 Classification of PH

PoPH is a type of precapillary PH. However, other forms of PH, such as PH due to left-sided heart disease, lung disease, and chronic hypoxemia, may coexist in chronic liver disease patients. So, understanding the other hemodynamic definition of PH is pertinent to the workup of PoPH.

Group 1: Pulmonary arterial hypertension (PAH). It includes Idiopathic PAH, POPH, connective tissue disease, HIV-associated PAH, congenital heart disease, and drug/toxin-induced PAH (Primarily precapillary).

Group 2 PH associated left-sided heart disease (both HF with preserved EF and reduced EF) Valvular heart disease (Primarily postcapillary).

Group 3 PH associated with lung disease and chronic hypoxia-related.

Group 4 Mostly includes chronic thromboembolic PH (CTEPH) (Primarily pre capillary).

Group 5 PH associated with the unclear or multifactorial mechanism.

3.5 Prevalence of PoPH

The prevalence of PoPH is assumed to be between 2% and 10% [29]. Up to 20% of patients undergoing LT have elevated pulmonary pressures; however, only 4% of patients have true PoPH [30]. More recent evidence shows the overall incidence of PH in patients undergoing LT is around 5.8%; of this, 73% are postcapillary PH, 14% PoPH, and 11.8% PH because of high cardiac output [31].

mPAP should not be used in isolation to characterize PoPH, as it does not define different pathological process. In cirrhosis PAP elevation may be caused by various chronic and/or acute pathological process and they have different management strategies and outcomes. Apart from primary pulmonary hypertension an increase in cardiac output (CO), left-to-right cardiac shunts, left heart disease (LHD), respiratory diseases, and various drugs may lead to elevated PAP [25]. Postcapillary PH is more common in CLD and it is characterized by elevated PAP and pulmonary artery wedge pressure (>15 mm Hg) and normal pulmonary vascular resistance (PVR) (<3 WU) [30]. This occurs due to volume overload because of secondary hyperaldosteronism and left ventricular dysfunction [32]. Unlike true PoPH, other types of PH do not seem to negatively affect the post-transplant outcome.

3.6 Screening and diagnosis

Dyspnea on exertion in the absence of gross ascites or pleural effusion, dyspnea when bending forward (Bendopnoea), chest pain, weakness, easy fatigability, peripheral edema, and syncope are symptoms of PoPH. However, these symptoms are common in chronic liver disease. On clinical examination jugular venous distension, an accentuated and split P2, right-sided S3 gallop, and right ventricular heave may hint towards PoPH. Electrocardiograms may display right axis deviation, right bundle branch block, and right ventricular strain. Chest radiographs may show enlarged right-sided chambers and dilatation of the pulmonary arteries. Pulmonary function tests may show decreased diffusion capacity, and the ventilation/perfusion lung scan is usually normal except in cases of chronic thromboembolic PH. Arterial blood gases (ABGs) may show an increased alveolar-arterial oxygen gradient (PA-a, O_2), mild-to-moderate hypoxemia, and decreased arterial carbon dioxide tension (<30 mm Hg) [27].

3.6.1 Transthoracic echocardiography

The single most important screening tool for PoPH is transthoracic echocardiography (TTE), and it is recommended in all patients getting evaluated for LT [33]. In the absence of right ventricular (RV) outflow tract obstruction, the RV systolic pressure (RVSP) estimated by tricuspid regurgitation velocity (TRV) is equal to pulmonary artery systolic pressure (PASP).

A PASP cut-off of >38 mm Hg was reported as the most accurate PASP cut off value to detect all forms of PoPH (specificity of 83%, negative predictive value of 100%). Diagnostic accuracy further increases by adding the presence of right ventricular dilatation to PASP cut-off (sensitivity of 100%, specificity of 93%, and negative predictive value of 100%) [34]. As only moderate to severe PoPH affect outcome post-transplant, liver transplant units have differed on when to investigate further with RHC. Mayo clinic suggesting PASP cut-off of 50 mm Hg whilst [35], The American Association for the Study of Liver Diseases (AASLD) has recommended a value of PASP >45 mm Hg [34].

Using the modified Bernoulli equation, PASP can be estimated from the tricuspid regurgitant jet velocity (TRV) [$PASP = 4V^2 +$ right atrial pressure (RAP)]. PASP measurement is considered the standard for estimating PAP [36]. However, in Bernoulli equation square of velocity is used so even a slight measurement error will get amplified, further RAP estimations are often inaccurate. Due to these two reasons, recent guidelines for pulmonary hypertension recommend using the peak TRV (>2.8 m/s) in place of estimated PASP, for the echocardiographic probability of PH [27].

Other echocardiography parameters which should be assessed alongside of PASP are measures of RV function, including the tricuspid annular plane systolic excursion (TAPSE), RV fractional area change (<35%), RV free-wall strain, and tricuspid annulus velocity (S′ wave). To differentiate between postcapillary (group 2) PH and other forms of PH both LV systolic function (LA size, LV hypertrophy, LV ejection fraction) and diastolic functions (e.g., E/A ratio, E/E′) should be assessed [27].

3.6.2 Right heat catheterization

Patients with liver disease frequently have volume overload and increased cardiac output, thus TRV tends to overestimate PASP. Hence, RHC is essential to confirm the diagnosis of PH and to distinguish true PoPH (with elevated PVR) from other types of PH (with a normal PVR). For a comprehensive assessment all measures listed in **Table 4** should be performed. All pressure measurements, including PAWP, should be taken at the end-expiration (without breath-holding manoeuvre) and should be averaged over at least three respiratory cycles [27].

Right atrial pressure, mean (RAP)
Pulmonary artery pressure, systolic (sPAP)
Pulmonary artery pressure, diastolic (dPAP)
Pulmonary artery pressure, mean (mPAP)
Pulmonary arterial wedge pressure, mean (PAWP)
Cardiac output (CO)
Pulmonary vascular resistance (PVR)
Mixed venous oxygen saturation (SvO2)
Systemic blood pressure

Table 4.
Parameters to be noted on RHC.

3.7 Differential diagnosis

PH is hemodynamically classified in precapillary PH, isolated postcapillary, and combined precapillary and postcapillary. As PH in chronic liver disease patients with multiple comorbidities can be due to PoPH or a combination of other precapillary and postcapillary causes it would be important to rule out a simple hyperdynamic state (PVR < 240 dynes/cm^5) or volume overload (PCWP >15 mm Hg), and more commonly postcapillary PH due to LV systolic or diastolic dysfunction. Some patients have elevated mPAP but low PVR and low PAWP. These patients do not fulfil the criteria for pre-, post-, or combined PH. This subgroup is described as unclassified PH and frequently characterized by elevated pulmonary blood flow which can be seen in patients with liver disease, airway disease, lung disease, or hyperthyroidism. Etiological workup for elevated pulmonary blood flow should be done [27] (**Table 5** showing differential diagnosis of PH in CLD).

3.8 Risk assessment

The severity of PoPH is based on resting mean PAP determined via RHC. It is graded as mild ($25 \leq$ mPAP < 35 mm Hg), moderate ($35 \leq$ mPAP <45 mm Hg), and severe (mPAP ≥ 45 mm Hg) [8].

		mPAP	**PVR**	**PAWP**	**CO**		**Probable patologies**
Diagnostic	POPH	↑	↑	↔	Mild ↑	Severe ↓	True POPH
Probable diagnosis	Hyperdynamic circulation and volume overload	↑	↔	↑	↑		Gross ascites AKI Albumin infusion
	PH with left heart disease	↑	↔	↑	HEpEF ↔	HFrEF ↓	Diastolic or Systolic dysfunction
	Unclassified PH	↑	↓	↓	↑↔↓		Congenital heart disease (CHD), liver disease, airway disease, lung disease, or hyperthyroidism

Table 5.
Hemodynamic pattern in chronic liver disease on right heart catheterization.

Signs of RV retrograde failure	Signs of RV forward failure
Distended and pulsating jugular vein	Peripheral cyanosis
Abdominal distension	Dizziness
Hepatomegaly	Pallor
Ascites	Cool extremities
Peripheral edema	Prolong capillary refill

Table 6.
Signs of right heart failure.

Baseline clinical assessment is an important benchmark for the assessment of disease severity and in determining whether it is improving, deteriorating, or getting stabilized. The appearance of physical signs of RV failure also indicates disease severity (Signs of RV failure enumerated in **Table 6**). The World Health Organization functional class (WHO-FC) at diagnosis and follow-up is one of the strongest predictors of survival [37], and worsening WHO-FC is an indicator of disease progression [38, 39]. According to estimated 1 year mortality and patients can be divided in to low, intermediate, and high risk. Other risk assessment parameters are pulmonary hemodynamics, 6-minute walk distance, biomarkers, and other echocardiographic parameters. (Risk assessment parameters are described in **Table** 7).

3.9 Pathophysiology and therapeutic targets

Medial hyperplasia, intimal proliferation and plexiform lesions formation leads to progressive pulmonary vasculopathy of PoPH. This vasculopathy leads to increase in pulmonary vascular resistance and gradual right ventricular failure. (**Figure 2** describe various pathophysiology and current therapeutic targets for PAH).

Patients with unclassified PH and isolated postcapillary PH should be followed up regularly, or liver transplant should be performed if there is significant liver dysfunction. They do not need PAH-specific therapy.

In patients with an established diagnosis of PoPH, PAH specific therapy should be started keeping following considerations:

- The severity of liver disease and urgency for LT
- PoPH specific indication and contraindication for LT.

PoPH patients are usually excluded from PAH treatment studies, but in principle, all drugs approved for PAH can be used to treat patients with PoPH. 5-year survival on PAH-specific therapy is 51% and reaches 81%, if patients underwent LT as well. In patients presenting with mild liver disease, the main causes of death were PAH progression and malignancy, whereas complications of liver disease were the most common causes of death in patients with advanced liver disease [40]. The only RCT dedicated to the treatment of PoPH, Macitentan, demonstrated a significant reduction in PVR from baseline [41].

3.10 Prognosis without LT

Analysis of a US registry data showed a median survival from time of diagnosis to be 27.5 months. Overall survival was 89%, 77%, 51%, and 38% at 6 months, 1 year, 3 years,

The prognosis (estimated 1-year mortality)	Low risk (<5%)	Intermediate risk (5–20%)	High risk (>20%)
Hemodynamics	RAP < 8 mm Hg	RAP 8–14 mm Hg	RAP > 14 mm Hg
	CI ⩾ 2.5 l/min/m^2	CI 2.0–2.4 l/min/m^2	CI < 2.0 l/min/m^2
	SVI > 38 ml/m^2	SVI 31–38 ml/m^2	SVI < 31 ml/m^2
	SvO2 > 65%	SvO2 60–65%	SvO2 < 60%
Signs of right HF	Absent	Absent	Present
History of syncope	No	Occasional[a]	Frequent[b]
Progression of symptoms and signs	No	Slow	Rapid
WHO-FC	I, II	III	IV
6 MWD	>440 m	165–440 m	<165 m
BNP	<50 ng/l	50–800 ng/l	>800 ng/l
NT-proBNP	<300 ng/l	300–1100 ng/l	>1100 ng/l
Echocardiography	RA area < 18 cm^2	RA area 18–26 cm^2	RA area > 26 cm^2
	TAPSE/PASP > 0.32 mm/mm Hg	TAPSE/PASP 0.19–0.32 mm/mm Hg	TAPSE/PASP <0.19 mm/mm Hg
	No pericardial effusion	Minimal pericardial effusion	Moderate or large pericardial effusion
cMRI	RVEF > 54%	RVEF 37–54%	RVEF < 37%
	SVI > 40 ml/m^2	SVI > 26–40 ml/m^2	SVI < 26 ml/m^2
	RVESVI<42 ml/m^2	RVESVI-2-54 ml/m^2	RVESVI>54 ml/m2

*6MWD, 6-minute walking distance; BNP, brain natriuretic peptide; CI, cardiac index; cMRI, cardiac magnetic resonance imaging; CPET, cardiopulmonary exercise testing; HF, heart failure; NT-proBNP, N-terminal pro-brain natriuretic peptide; PAH, pulmonary arterial hypertension; pred., predicted; RA, right atrium; RAP, right atrial pressure; sPAP, systolic pulmonary arterial pressure; SvO2, mixed venous oxygen saturation; RVESVI, right ventricular end-systolic volume index; RVEF, right ventricular ejection fraction; SVI, stroke volume index; TAPSE, tricuspid annular plane systolic excursion; WHO-FC, World Health Organization functional class. Adapted and reproduced with permission of the © European Society of Cardiology & European Respiratory Society 2023: European Respiratory Journal **61**(1):2200879; DOI: 10.1183/13993003.00879-2022. Published 6 January 2023 (from Ref. [28]).*
[a]Occasional syncope during heavy exercise or occasional orthostatic syncope in a stable patient.[b]Repeated episodes of syncope even with little or regular physical activity.

Table 7.
Risk assessment in pulmonary artery hypertension.

and 5 years, respectively. Patients with PoPH who did not undergo LT had a poor prognosis [27]. United Kingdom National Pulmonary Hypertension Service registry reported 3-year survival of 60% and survival of patients with PoPH remained poor despite targeted therapy and worse than patients with idiopathic PAH [42]. However, in both studies, most of the patients were on monotherapy and recent use of combination therapy has shown improved outcomes (3- and 5-year survival, 88.5% and 80.2%, respectively) [43].

3.11 Liver transplantation and prognosis after LT

Postcapillary PH does not negatively affect post-liver transplant survival, and a higher cardiac output (11 l/min in patients who lived, as compared with 8 l/min in

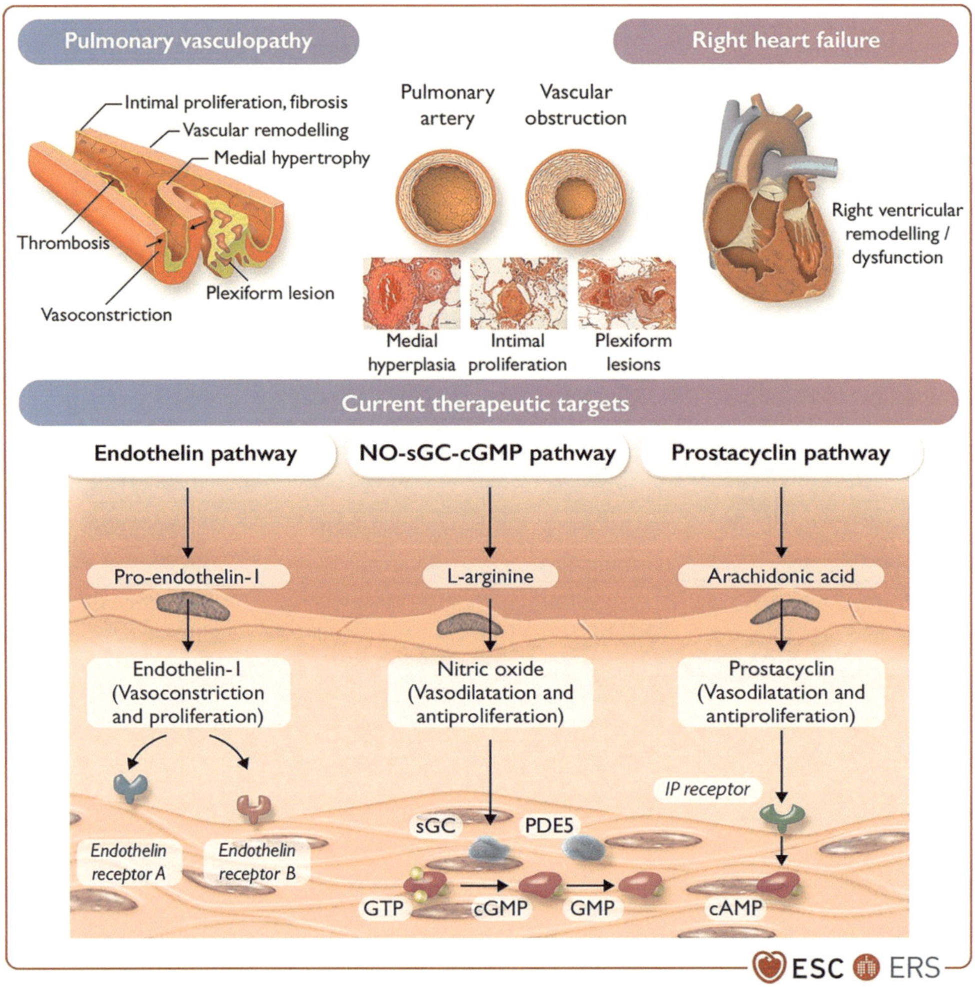

Figure 2.
Pathophysiology and current therapeutic targets of pulmonary arterial hypertension (group 1). cAMP, cyclic adenosine monophosphate; (c)GMP, (cyclic) guanosine monophosphate; GTP, guanosine-5'-triphosphate; IP receptor, prostacyclin I2 receptor; NO, nitric oxide; PDE5, phosphodiesterase 5; sGC, soluble guanylate cyclase. Reproduced with permission of the © European Society of Cardiology & European Respiratory Society 2023: European Respiratory Journal ***61*** *(1):2200879; DOI: 10.1183/13993003.00879-2022. Published 6 January 2023 (from Ref. [28]).*

patients who died) may be protective against mortality in patients with postcapillary PH [30]. Mortality rate after LT according to severity stood 100%, 50%, and 0% in patients with mPAP >50 mm Hg, 35–50 mm Hg, and <35 mm Hg, respectively [44]. Patients in whom mPAP was ≤35 mm Hg, both the graft and patient survival rates were found to be 85.7% after a median follow-up of 7.8 years [45]. Achieving reduction in PVR < 250 dynes/s per cm^{-5} by PAH specific therapy, even if mPAP remains ≥35 mm Hg before LT has shown 69% 1-year post-transplant survival and PAH specific therapy can be discontinued in majority of patients [46]. This shows importance of reduction of PVR before proceeding for LT.

Patients with mild PoPH do not possess an increased risk for LT, so they should be considered for LT. Patients with an mPAP between 35 and 45 mm Hg should undergo PAH-specific treatment, and who reach a reduction of mPAP to ≤35 mm Hg and PVR

<400 dynes/s per cm^{-5} should be offered LT [34]. The ILTS practice guideline further added LT could also be considered if treated PoPH does not reduce mPAP to <35 mm Hg, but there is a normalization of PVR (<240 dynes/s per cm^{-5}), as it does not seems to be associated with adverse outcomes [13].

4. Hepatic hydrothorax

A transudative pleural effusion in a patient with chronic liver disease with portal hypertension or cirrhosis in the absence of other etiological factors is termed hepatic hydrothorax (HH) [47]. A median survival of 8–12 months is reported once it is diagnosed [48].

Usually, ascites is a precursor of hydrothorax. Ascites coexists in 80% of cases but are not mandatory for diagnosis [49]. The hypothesis based on the trans-diaphragmatic shift of fluid vial defects in the diaphragm is commonly accepted and this theory is endorsed by evidence of macro- and microscopic diaphragmatic defects [50]. HH has a predilection for the right side as the right diaphragm is thinner and less muscular with frequent defects as compared to the left. Radiolabelled 99mTc-sulfur colloid or 99mTc-albumin transmigration from the peritoneal to the pleural cavity has been demonstrated earlier to support the theory [51]. As per the studies, overall, the prevalence is 70% right sides, 18% bilateral, and 12% left-sided HH [52]. In HH with ascites, negative intrathoracic pressures in during inspiration promotes fluid accumulation in the pleural space [53].

Patients usually present with severe but nonspecific complaints of dyspnoea at rest (4%), dyspnoea on exertion (7%), non-productive cough (22%), pleuritic chest pain (8%), dizziness or fatigue (7%). In extreme cases, respiratory failure and subsequent heart failure is also reported [54]. Once established on radiological evidence, the nature of effusion (exudative or transudative) is determined by diagnostic thoracocentesis.

HH is characterized by a total cell count of polymorphonucleocytes <250/µl, a total protein concentration < 2.5 g/dl, a serum to pleural albumin gradient >1.1 g/dl, or a pleural fluid to serum albumin quotient <0.6. Other parameters indicating HH are an LDH gradient <0.6 (serum—pleural fluid) and similar pH value, as well as glucose concentration in serum and pleural fluid [55]. Other supportive investigations are to be performed to rule out the differentials in consideration, including pleural effusion of other etiology, pancreatitis, thoracic or abdominal malignancies, etc. complimentary abdominal sonography is helpful in diagnosis or prognostication of already diagnosed underlying CLD.

The treatment principle of treatment is essentially on parallel lines with that of the treatment of ascites, which includes sodium restriction, diuresis, and large-volume paracentesis for respiratory insufficiency. The invasive procedure of therapeutic thoracocentesis should be performed only if symptoms persist. Precautions in the form of pleural puncture volume up to 2 l/Puncture, and substitution of 6–8 gm albumin/litre can be taken to avoid re-expansion pulmonary edema. Continuous thoracic drainage is not recommended in view of the loss of proteins and increased rate of infections [56].

Trans-jugular intrahepatic portosystemic shunt (TIPS) may be beneficial for rare intractable cases. Attempts in reduction of portal hypertension, the recovery was seen in 56% and improvement in 18% [57]. Pleurodesis may be performed; having said that, it has a high relapse of 25% and complications in 80% [58]. Surgical treatment in the form of pleural flaps or mesh reinforcement has been described [59].

Refractory hepatic hydrothorax (RHH) is defined by the failure to control symptomatic HH with sodium restriction (<2 g/day), tolerable amounts of diuretic (160 mg/day furosemide and 400 mg/day spironolactone, or repeated thoracentesis) [60].

Liver transplantation is the only curative therapeutic option [61]. The patients with preoperative HH have higher rates of postoperative infections, emphasizing the relevance of HH as an adverse prognostic factor [62]. HH persisted in one-third of patients till 1-month post-LT but resolved completely in all patients within 3 months of transplant [63].

5. Spontaneous bacterial empyema

Analogous to spontaneous bacterial peritonitis, spontaneous bacterial empyema (SBE) is a specific complication of HH [64]. The overall prevalence of SBE is 2.4% of CLDs, the incidence increases to 10–16% in the decompensated state of HH, and the mortality associated with SBE is 38% [65]. Half of the patients with concomitant HH and SBP develop SBE [66]. Pleural fluid examination typically suggests low total proteins and albumin, C3 compliments [67, 68].

The patient may present with nonspecific symptoms and sometimes with worsening in liver function. The diagnosis should be based on thoracocentesis with a total polymorphonucleocytes >250/microlitres with cultures growing the organisms or >500 per microlitres with no growth on culture. The most common organisms growing are *Escherichia coli*, Klebsiella, Streptococcus, or Enterococcus. Although 2/3rd of the patients remains culture negative and most of the patients have a history of multiple hospital admissions, such are at risk of multidrug-resistant bacteria [69, 70].

The treatment consists of intravenous antibiotics as per local antibiogram immediately after the pleural fluid sampling [21]. Streptokinase and, in extreme, video-assisted thoracoscopic surgery may be the only options [71].

6. Restrictive lung disease

Restrictive lung diseases are group of varied lung disorders defined by restrictive patterns (forced vital capacity (FVC) <70% predicted) on spirometry. Restrictive lung diseases may be caused by intrinsic conditions (interstitial lung disease, ILD) or by extrinsic conditions (limitations in neuromuscular function and chest wall movements, obesity). In CLD prevalence of restrictive lung disease is 18.4%, and it is associated with lower 6-minute walk distances, dyspnea, worse quality of life, and increased risk of death [72]. Restrictive abnormalities correlate with prolonged after LT ventilation and length of stay. Efforts to identify and minimize the impact of restrictive abnormalities on PFTs might improve outcomes [73].

ILD defines progressive inflammatory and fibrotic diseases targeting the pulmonary interstitial tissue. It has an affinity to be associated with primary biliary cirrhosis, autoimmune hepatitis, or hepatitis [74]. It leads to progressive hypoxemia and may contribute to hypoxia caused by HPS [75]. 99mTcMAA lung perfusion scan can differentiate between ILD and HPS as brain uptake is normal (<6%) in ILD. Patients with ILD characteristically have a restrictive pattern and a decrease in DLCO. The most common radiographic feature observed is a reticular pattern. However, nodular or mixed patterns can be seen. High-resolution computed tomography

(HRCT) shows coarse crosslinking in basal regions in early stage and honeycombing in later stages. LT should be avoided in moderate to severe restrictive lung disease due to ILD [76].

7. Asthma and chronic obstructive pulmonary disease (COPD)

Asthma is a reversible airway obstructive disease with bronchial hyperreactivity. There is no evidence regarding the influence of asthma on outcomes after liver transplant.

COPD is a progressive lung disease characterized by non-reversible airflow limitation caused by chronic inflammation and mucus hypersecretion. Severity classification done on basis of FEV1% predicted. For mild COPD FEV1% predicted ≥80%, moderate as FEV1% predicted ≥50% and <80%, severe as FEV1% predicted ≥30% and <50% and very severe as FEV1% predicted <30% [77]. Around 18% of new patients undergoing LT evaluation have COPD particularly if they are older and have history of smoking. 80% patients had the diagnosis of COPD made for the first time during their LT evaluation. Despite the impact of COPD on functional status and quality of life, the risk of death and post-LT outcomes were not affected by the existence or severity of COPD [78]. However, in this study, only 11% of patients had severe COPD (30% < FEV1% predicted <50%), and no patient had FEV1% < 30%. Long-term post-LT outcomes in COPD are poorly characterized. Very severe COPD should be considered a contraindication for LT, and in severe COPD, detailed evaluation and risk stratification should be done before considering LT.

8. Conclusion

HPS and POPH are pulmonary complications of liver disease and portal hypertension. All pulmonary manifestations of liver disease, except uncontrolled moderate and Severe POPH, are treatable with liver transplantation with a good outcome. LT not only halts the progression of these diseases but also leads to complete resolution. As both CLD-specific pulmonary disorders and chronic liver disease in itself are progressive diseases, the gradual worsening of both has a dual, negative effect on the outcome. The increasing severity of these pulmonary manifestations increases waitlist mortality and inferior survival after liver transplants. Early identification and optimization of these manifestations and the timely liver transplant are reasonable. Dyspnea on exertion and sometimes at rest is a common index symptom of respiratory insufficiency; however, in liver disease due to ascites, pleural effusion, poor nutrition, sarcopenia, and chronic illness, dyspnea is otherwise a very common presentation. So high index of suspicion is required in CLD for asymptomatic as well as symptomatic respiratory symptoms. The approach must focus on determining whether the etiology is pre-existing, CLD-specific (HPS, POPH), or a combination of both. The accurate identification of the primary pulmonary issue, quantifying its severity, and assessment of additional abnormalities becomes important for patients' symptomatic treatment, optimization before transplantation, and perioperative management.

Conflict of interest

The authors declare no conflict of interest.

Author details

Vijay Kant Pandey[1*], Aaditya Anil Prabhudesai[2] and Subhash Gupta[1]

1 Center for Liver and Biliary Sciences, Max Super Specialty Hospital, New Delhi, India

2 Liver Anesthesia and Critical Care, Nanavati Max Super Specialty Hospital, Mumbai, India

*Address all correspondence to: drvijay17@gmail.com

References

[1] Fuhrmann V, Krowka M. Hepatopulmonary syndrome. Journal of Hepatology. 2018;**69**(3):744-745

[2] Fallon MB, Krowka MJ, Brown RS, Trotter JF, Zacks S, Roberts KE, et al. Impact of hepatopulmonary syndrome on quality of life and survival in liver transplant candidates. Gastroenterology. 2008;**135**(4):1168-1175. DOI: 10.1053/j.gastro.2008.06.038

[3] Gupta S, Castel H, Rao RV. Improved survival after liver transplantation in patients with hepatopulmonary syndrome. American Journal of Transplantation. 2010;**10**(2):354-363. DOI: 10.1111/j.1600-6143.2009.02822.x. Epub 2009 Sep 22

[4] Machicao VI, Balakrishnan M, Fallon MB. Pulmonary complications in chronic liver disease. Hepatology. 2014;**59**:1627-1637. DOI: 10.1002/hep.26745

[5] Arguedas M, Singh H, Faulk D. Utility of pulse oximetry screening for hepatopulmonary syndrome. Clinical Gastroenterology and Hepatology. 2007;**5**:749-754

[6] Hoerning A, Raub S, Neudorf U. Pulse oximetry is insufficient for timely diagnosis of hepatopulmonary syndrome in children with liver cirrhosis. The Journal of Pediatrics. 2014;**164**:546-552

[7] Forde KA, Fallon MB, Krowka MJ, Sprys M, Goldberg DS, Krok KL, et al. Pulse oximetry is insensitive for detection of hepatopulmonary syndrome in patients evaluated for liver transplantation. Hepatology. 2016;**69**:270-281. DOI: 10.1002/hep.30139

[8] Rodriguez-Roisin R, Krowka MJ, Herve P. Pulmonary-hepatic vascular disorders (PHD). The European Respiratory Journal. 2004;**24**:861-880. DOI: 10.1097/TP.0000000000001229 Same is adapted by ILTS

[9] Bommena S, Gerkin RD, Agarwal S, Raevens S, Glassberg MK, Fallon MB. Diagnosis of hepatopulmonary syndrome in a large integrated health system. Clinical Gastroenterology and Hepatology. 2021;**19**:2370-2378. DOI: 10.1016/j.cgh.2020.09.050. Epub 2020 Sep 30. PMID: 33007510

[10] Krowka MJ, Dickson ER, Cortese DA. Hepatopulmonary syndrome. Clinical observations and lack of therapeutic response to somatostatin analogue. Chest. 1993;**104**:515-521. DOI: 10.1378/chest.104.2.515 PMID: 8101797

[11] Luo B-W, Du Z-Y. Advances in diagnostic imaging of Hepatopulmonary syndrome. Frontiers in Medicine. 2022;**8**:817758. DOI: 10.3389/fmed.2021.817758

[12] Krowka MJ, Fallon MB, Kawut SM, Fuhrmann V, Heimbach JK, Ramsay MA, et al. International liver transplant society practice guidelines: Diagnosis and management of hepatopulmonary syndrome and portopulmonary hypertension. Transplantation. 2016;**100**(7):1440-1452. DOI: 10.1097/TP.0000000000001229

[13] El-Shabrawi MH, Omran S, Wageeh S. 99mTechnetium-macroaggregated albumin perfusion lung scan versus contrast enhanced echocardiography in the diagnosis of the hepatopulmonary syndrome in children with chronic liver disease. European Journal of Gastroenterology & Hepatology. 2010;**22**:1006-1012

[14] Zhao H, Tsauo J, Zhang XW, Ma HY, Weng NN, Tang GS, et al. Technetium-

99m-labeled macroaggregated albumin lung perfusion scan for diagnosis of hepatopulmonary syndrome: A prospective study comparing brain uptake and whole-body uptake. World Journal of Gastroenterology. 2020; **26**(10):1088-1097. DOI: 10.3748/wjg.v26.i10.1088 PMID: 32205999; PMCID: PMC7080996

[15] Raevens S, Boret M, Fallon MB. Hepatopulmonary syndrome. JHEP Reports. 2022;**4**(4):100527. DOI: 10.1016/j.jhepr.2022.100527 PMID: 36035361; PMCID: PMC9403489

[16] Raevens S, Fallon MB. Potential clinical targets in hepatopulmonary syndrome: Lessons from experimental models. Hepatology. 2018;**68**:2016-2028. DOI: 10.1002/hep.30079

[17] Van Thiel DH, Schade RR, Gavaler JS. Medical aspects of liver transplantation. Hepatology. 1984;**4**: 79S-83S

[18] Goldberg D, Olthof K. Standardizing MELD exceptions: Current challenges and future directions. Current Transplantation Reports. 2014;**1**:232-237. DOI: 10.1007/s40472-014-0027-4

[19] Swanson KL, Wiesner RH, Krowka MJ. Natural history of hepatopulmonary syndrome: Impact of liver transplantation. Hepatology. 2005; **41**:1122-1129. DOI: 10.1002/hep.20658

[20] Goldberg DS, Krok K, Batra S. Impact of the hepatopulmonary syndrome MELD exception policy on outcomes of patients after liver transplantation: An analysis of the UNOS database. Gastroenterology. 2014;**146**: 1256-1265

[21] Kadry Z, Schaefer E, Krok K, Faust A, Stine JG, Schreibman IR, et al. Excellent outcomes with liver transplantation in hepatopulmonary syndrome across pre-transplant PaO2 spectrum. JHEP Reports. 2021;**3**:100351. DOI: 10.1016/j.jhepr.2021.100351 PMID: 34604726; PMCID: PMC8473556

[22] Fauconnet P, Klopfenstein CE, Schiffer E. Hepatopulmonary syndrome: The anaesthetic considerations. European Journal of Anaesthesiology. 2013;**30**:721-730

[23] Nayyar D, Man H.S.J, Granton J, Gupta, S. Defining and characterizing severe hypoxemia after liver transplantation in hepatopulmonary syndrome. Liver Transplantation 2004; 20: 182-190. DOI:10.1002/lt.23776.

[24] Kelly Wu W, Grogan WM, Ziogas IA, Patel YJ, Bacchetta M, Alexopoulos SP. Extracorporeal membrane oxygenation in patients with hepatopulmonary syndrome undergoing liver transplantation: A systematic review of the literature. Transplantation Reviews 2022;36:100693. ISSN 0955-470X, DOI:10.1016/j.trre.2022.100693.

[25] Hatano S, Strasser T. Primary pulmonary hypertension. In: Report on a WHO Meeting. Geneva: World Health Organization; 1975

[26] Simonneau G, Montani D, Celermajer DS. Haemodynamic definitions and updated clinical classification of pulmonary hypertension. The European Respiratory Journal. 2019;**53**:1801913. DOI: 10.1183/13993003.01913-2018

[27] Kovacs G, Berghold A, Scheidl S, Olschewski H. Pulmonary arterial pressure during rest and exercise in healthy subjects: A systematic review. The European Respiratory Journal. 2009; **34**:888-894. DOI: 10.1183/09031936.00145608

[28] Humbert M, Kovacs G, Hoeper MM. 2022 ESC/ERS Guidelines for the diagnosis and treatment of pulmonary hypertension. The European Respiratory Journal. 2023;**61**:2200879. DOI: 10.1183/13993003.00879-2022

[29] Hadengue A, Benhayoun MK, Lebrec D, Benhamou JP. Pulmonary hypertension complicating portal hypertension: Prevalence and relation to splanchnic hemodynamics. Gastroenterology. 1991;**100**(2):520-528

[30] Castro M, Krowka MJ, Schroeder DR, Beck KC, Plevak DJ, Rettke SR, et al. Frequency and clinical implications of increased pulmonary artery pressures in liver transplant patients. Mayo Clinic Proceedings. 1996; **71**(6):543-551. DOI: 10.4065/71.6.543 PMID: 8642882

[31] Cerise K, Aggarwal M, Tonelli AR, White M, Lyu R, Quintini C, et al. Liver transplant outcomes in patients with postcapillary pulmonary hypertension. Transplantation direct. 2022;**8**(11):e1372 | DOI: 10.1097/TXD.0000000000001372

[32] Møller S, Henriksen JH. Cirrhotic cardiomyopathy: A pathophysiological review of circulatory dysfunction in liver disease. Heart. 2002;**87**:9-15

[33] Martin P, DiMartini A, Feng S, Brown R Jr, Fallon M. Evaluation for liver transplantation in adults: 2013 practice guideline by the American Association for the Study of Liver Diseases and the American Society of Transplantation. Hepatology. 2014; **59**(3):1144-1165. DOI: 10.1002/hep.26972

[34] Raevens S, Colle I, Reyntjens K, Geerts A, Berrevoet F, Rogiers X, et al. Echocardiography for the detection of portopulmonary hypertension in liver transplant candidates: An analysis of cutoff values. Liver Transplantation. 2013;**19**:602-610. DOI: 10.1002/lt.23649

[35] Kim WR, Krowka MJ, Plevak DJ, Lee J, Rettke SR, Frantz RP, Wiesner R. H. Accuracy of doppler echocardiography in the assessment of pulmonary hypertension in liver transplant candidates. Liver Transplantation, 2000;6: 453-458. doi: 10.1053/jlts.2000.7573

[36] Armstrong DW, Tsimiklis G, Matangi MF. Factors influencing the echocardiographic estimate of right ventricular systolic pressure in normal patients and clinically relevant ranges according to age. The Canadian Journal of Cardiology. 2010;**26**(2):e35-e39

[37] Barst RJ, Chung L, Zamanian RT. Functional class improvement and 3-year survival outcomes in patients with pulmonary arterial hypertension in the REVEAL Registry. Chest. 2013;**144**: 160-168

[38] Barst RJ, Chung L, Zamanian RT. Functional class improvement and 3-year survival outcomes in patients with pulmonary arterial hypertension in the REVEAL Registry. Chest. 2013;**144**: 160-168, 210, 213, 214

[39] Humbert M, Sitbon O, Yaici A. Survival in incident and prevalent cohorts of patients with pulmonary arterial hypertension. The European Respiratory Journal. 2010;**36**:549-555

[40] Savale L, Guimas M, Ebstein N. Portopulmonary hypertension in the current era of pulmonary hypertension management. Journal of Hepatology. 2020;**73**:130-139

[41] Sitbon O, Bosch J, Cottreel E, Csonka D, de Groote P, Hoeper MM. Macitentan for the treatment of portopulmonary hypertension

(PORTICO): A multicentre, randomised, doubleblind, placebo-controlled, phase 4 trial. The Lancet Respiratory Medicine. 2019;7:594e604

[42] Sithamparanathan S, Nair A, Thirugnanasothy L. Survival in portopulmonary hypertension: Outcomes of the United Kingdom National Pulmonary Arterial hypertension Registry. The Journal of Heart and Lung Transplantation. 2017;**36**:770-779. DOI: 10.1016/j.healun.2016.12.014

[43] Tamura Y, Tamura Y, Taniguchi Y. Clinical management and outcomes of patients with portopulmonary hypertension enrolled in the Japanese Multicenter Registry. Circulation Reports. 2022;**4**:542-549. DOI: 10.1253/circrep.CR-22-0098

[44] Krowka MJ, Plevak DJ, Findlay JY, Rosen CB, Wiesner RH, Krom RAF. Pulmonary hemodynamics and perioperative cardiopulmonary-related mortality in patients with portopulmonary hypertension undergoing liver transplantation. Liver Transplantation. 2000;**6**:443-450

[45] Khaderi S, Khan R, Safdar Z, Stribling R, Vierling JM, Goss JA, et al. Long-term follow-up of portopulmonary hypertension patients after liver transplantation. Liver Transplantation. 2014;**20**:724-727. DOI: 10.1002/lt.23870

[46] DuBrock HM, Runo JR, Sadd CJ, Burger CD, Cartin-Ceba R, Rosen CB, et al. Outcomes of liver transplantation in treated portopulmonary hypertension patients with a mean pulmonary arterial pressure ≥35 mmHg. Transplantation direct. 2020;**6**:e630. DOI: 10.1097/TXD.0000000000001085

[47] Krok KL. Hepatic hydrothorax: Current concepts. Clinics in Liver Disease. 2014;**4**:35-37

[48] Badillo R, Rockey DC. Hepatic hydrothorax: Clinical features, management, and outcomes in 77 patients and review of the literature. Medicine. 2014;**93**:135-142

[49] Gurung P, Goldblatt M, Huggins JT, Doelken P, Nietert PJ, Sahn SA. Pleural fluid analysis and radiographic, sonographic, and echocardiographic characteristics of hepatic hydrothorax. Chest. 2011;**140**:448-453

[50] Huang PM, Chang YL, Yang CY, Lee YC. The morphology of diaphragmatic defects in hepatic hydrothorax: Thoracoscopic finding. The Journal of Thoracic and Cardiovascular Surgery. 2005;**130**:141-145

[51] Bhattacharya A, Mittal BR, Biswas T, Dhiman RK, Singh B, Jindal SK. Radioisotope scintigraphy in the diagnosis of hepatic hydrothorax. Journal of Gastroenterology and Hepatology. 2001;**16**:317-321

[52] Malagari K, Nikita A, Alexopoulou E, Brountzos E, Papathanasiou M, Mitromaras J, et al. Imaging features in 1038 patients. Hepato-Gastroenterology. 2005;**52**:558-562

[53] Benz F, Mohr R, Tacke F, Roderburg C. Pulmonary complications in patients with liver cirrhosis. Journal of Translational Internal Medicine. 2020;**8**:150-158

[54] Light RW. Clinical practice. Pleural effusion. The New England Journal of Medicine. 2002;**346**:1971-1977

[55] Singh A, Bajwa A, Shujaat A. Evidence-based review of the management of hepatic hydrothorax. Respiration. 2013;**86**:155-173

[56] Liu LU, Haddadin HA, Bodian CA, Sigal SH, Korman JD, Bodenheimer HC.

Outcome analysis of cirrhotic patients undergoing chest tube placement. Chest. 2004;**126**:142-148

[57] Ditah IC, Al Bawardy BF, Saberi B, Ditah C, Kamath PS. Transjugular intrahepatic portosystemic stent shunt for medically refractory hepatic hydrothorax: A systematic review and cumulative meta-analysis. World Journal of Hepatology. 2015;7:1797-1806

[58] Hou F, Qi X, Guo X. Effectiveness and safety of pleurodesis for hepatic hydrothorax: A systematic review and meta-analysis. Digestive Diseases and Sciences. 2016;**61**:3321-3334

[59] Huang PM, Kuo SW, Chen JS, Lee JM. Thoracoscopic mesh repair of diaphragmatic defects in hepatic hydrothorax: A 10-year experience. The Annals of Thoracic Surgery. 2016;**101**: 1921-1927

[60] Krok KL, Cardenas A. Hepatic hydrothorax. Seminars in Respiratory and Critical Care Medicine. 2012;**33**:3-10

[61] Sersté TD, Moreno C, Francoz C, Razek WA, Paugham C, Belghitti J, et al. The impact of preoperative hepatic hydrothorax on the outcome of adult liver transplantation. European Journal of Gastroenterology & Hepatology. 2010;**22**:207-212. DOI: 10.1097/MEG.0b013e3283311140

[62] Endo K, Iida T, Yagi S, Yoshizawa A, Fujimoto Y, Ogawa K. Impact of preoperative uncontrollable hepatic hydrothorax and massive ascites in adult liver transplantation. Surgery Today. 2014;**44**:2293-2299

[63] Xiol X, Tremosa G, Castellote J, Gornals J, Lama C, Lopez C. Liver transplantation in patients with hepatic hydrothorax. Transplant International. 2005;**18**:672-675

[64] Tu CY, Chen CH. Spontaneous bacterial empyema. Current Opinion in Pulmonary Medicine. 2012;**18**:355-358

[65] Chen CH, Shih CM, Chou JW, Liu YH, Hang LW, Hsia TC. Outcome predictors of cirrhotic patients with spontaneous bacterial empyema. Liver International. 2011;**31**:417-424

[66] Ewig S, Hoffken G, Kern WV, Rohde G, Flick H, Krause R. Management of adult community-acquired pneumonia and prevention—Update 2016. Pneumologie. 2016;**70**: 151-200

[67] Ackerman Z, Reynolds TB. Evaluation of pleural fluid in patients with cirrhosis. Journal of Clinical Gastroenterology. 1997;**25**:619-622

[68] Sese E, Xiol X, Castellote J, Rodriguez-Farinas E, Tremosa G. Low complement levels and opsonic activity in hepatic hydrothorax: Its relationship with spontaneous bacterial empyema. Journal of Clinical Gastroenterology. 2003;**36**:75-77

[69] Fernández J, Prado V, Trebicka J, Amoros A, Gustot T, Wiest R. Multidrug-resistant bacterial infections in patients with decompensated cirrhosis and with acute-on-chronic liver failure in Europe. Journal of Hepatology. 2019; **70**:398-411

[70] Piano S, Singh V, Caraceni P, Maiwall R, Alessandria C, Fernandez J. Epidemiology and effects of bacterial infections in patients with cirrhosis worldwide. Gastroenterology. 2019;**156**: 1368-80.e1310

[71] Xiol X, Castellvi JM, Guardiola J, Sese E, Castellote J, Perello A. Spontaneous bacterial empyema in cirrhotic patients: A prospective study. Hepatology. 1996;**23**:719-723

[72] DuBrock HM, Krowka MJ, Krok K, Forde K, Mottram C, Scanlon P, et al. Prevalence and impact of restrictive lung disease in liver transplant candidates. Liver Transplantation. 2020;**26**:989-999. DOI: 10.1002/lt.25794

[73] Kia L, Cuttica MJ, Yang A. The utility of pulmonary function testing in predicting outcomes following liver transplantation. Liver Transplantation. 2016;**22**(6):805-811. DOI: 10.1002/lt.24426

[74] Spagnolo PC, Zeuzem S, Richeldi L, Du Bois RM. The complex interrelationships between chronic lung and liver disease: A review. Journal of Viral Hepatitis. 2010;**17**:381-390. DOI: 10.1111/j.1365-2893.2010.01307.x

[75] Martinez G, Barbera JA, Navasa M, Roca J, Visa J, Rodriguez-Roisin R. Hepatopulmonary syndrome associated with cardiorespiratory disease. Journal of Hepatology. 1999;**30**:882-889

[76] Krowka MJ, Wiesner RH, Heimbach JK. Pulmonary contraindications, indications and MELD exceptions for liver transplantation: A contemporary view and look forward. Journal of Hepatology. 2013;**59**:367-374. DOI: 10.1016/j.jhep.2013.03.026

[77] Rabe KF, Hurd S, Anzueto A, Barnes PJ, Buist SA, Calverey P. Global strategy for the diagnosis, management, and prevention of chronic obstructive pulmonary disease: GOLD executive summary. American Journal of Respiratory and Critical Care Medicine. 2007;**176**:532-555

[78] Rybak D, Fallon MB, Krowka MJ, Brown RS Jr, Reinen J, Stadheim L, et al. Risk factors and impact of chronic obstructive pulmonary disease in candidates for liver transplantation. Liver Transplantation. 2008;**14**: 1357-1365. DOI: 10.1002/lt.21545

Chapter 6

Mechanical Ventilation in the Burn Patient

José Manuel Araiza-Sanchez, Pedro Yasfir González-Noris, Juan José Espinoza-Espinosa and Marcos Alfonso Rosas

Abstract

Among the most difficult to treat are severely burned, patients. We examined the conditions of these patients individually and the organ involvement. It is impossible to manage them because they are dealing with multi-organ dysfunction, which affects all system homeostasis. This chapter focuses on the respiratory system, specifically the mechanical ventilation strategies to improve the outcome in the onset of acute respiratory distress syndrome (ARDS) and inhalation injury in severely burned patients, beginning with initial airway management and progressing to new ventilation strategies and modes to assist health providers in choosing what is best for their patients.

Keywords: severely burned, ARDS, protective ventilation, inhalation injury, carbon monoxide

1. Introduction

Making the decision to act before ARDS develops is one of the most difficult challenges in the management of severely burned patients. The Abbreviated Burn Severity Index (ABSI) and the modern modified ABSI are two predictors of the development of ARDS in burn patients [1, 2]. We can improve the survival rate and the number of ventilator-free days for burn patients by acting quickly in the airway and ventilator management.

With the development of lung-protective ventilation and the Berlin Criteria for the diagnosis and classification of ARDS, mechanical ventilation management has improved dramatically in recent years [3], and we now rely on new ventilation methods with promising results when it comes to improving ARDS outcomes.

This chapter will focus on the mechanisms of how ARDS develops in severely burned patients, from the chemical foundation to the physical and macroscopic injuries a burned airway must endure.

2. Initial airway management

Airway assessment and cervical spine immobilization are the first steps in the management of severely burn patients, as they are in severe trauma. Burns to the upper and lower airways, as well as inhalation injury (II), pose a higher risk of airway obstruction. Therefore, early recognition of the signs and symptoms indicating the need for advanced airway management is critical.

According to the current trend in difficult airway management, it is preferable to have a team to minimize the complication rate in critical scenarios. Anesthesiologists, trauma surgeons, and head and neck surgeons are typically part of this team.

Burn patients have a difficult airway due to airway edema, the need for cervical protection, and the friability of the airway mucosa (**Figure 1**). Thus, it is recommended that the intubation be performed by an airway expert to avoid the need for a surgical airway and further complications [4].

According to Advanced Trauma Life Support, the following are indications for early intubation:

- Signs of airway obstruction
- Total body surface area burns of >40%
- Deep facial burns or burns inside the mouth
- Edema or risk for edema

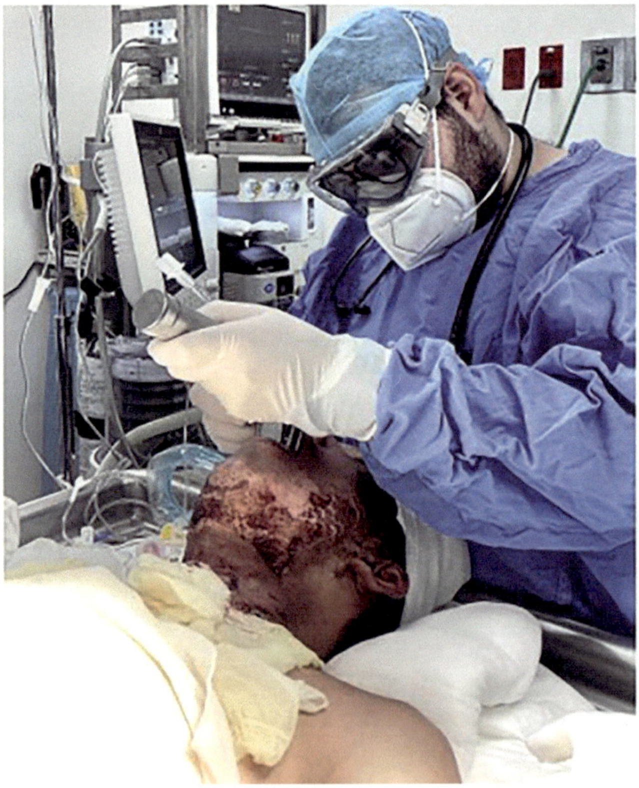

Figure 1.
Manuel Araiza managing a severely burned patient airway, in May 2022; notice the neck burns and the airway positioning to stabilize cervical spine, which are included in the difficult airways characteristics.

- Difficulty swallowing
- Signs of respiratory compromise
- Low level of consciousness, impairment of the airway protective reflexes, and
- Management of unqualified personnel

Rapid sequence intubation (RSI) is the technique of choice for advanced airway management in severely burned patients to minimize the risk of regurgitation and optimize oxygen delivery. Rocuronium and suxamethonium are two neuromuscular blockers used in RSI. Suxamethonium increases the risk of hyperkalemia, bradycardia, high intracranial pressure, high intraocular pressure, and fasciculations [5], so its use in advanced airway management in burn patients should be limited.

3. Carbon monoxide and hydrogen cyanide toxicity

3.1 Carbon monoxide toxicity

Incomplete combustion produces carbon monoxide (CO) as a by-product. It is very common to find exposure to this chemical when inhalation injury is present, as it is odorless and tasteless. The main problem with CO poisoning is the wide range of symptoms it can cause: from a mild headache to seizures and death. Therefore, in all severely burned patients, we should always suspect and assess for CO poisoning.

CO inhibits the release of oxygen into peripheral tissues, resulting in tissue hypoxia. However, the molecular mechanisms are more complex.

The binding of CO to intracellular proteins such as cytochromes, myoglobin, and guanylyl cyclase disrupts cell homeostasis, interferes with oxidative metabolism, promotes the formation of reactive oxygen species, and causes oxidative stress and cell apoptosis [6].

Assessing for CO poisoning using the carboxyhemoglobin (COHb) measurement can provide insight into the severity of the intoxication, but COHb levels do not always correlate with the degree of poisoning [6]. It has been classically stated that COHb levels of 15–40% can cause moderate symptoms, and levels of >40% can cause severe symptoms and death from CO toxicity [4].

CO poisoning symptoms are classified into three levels: mild, moderate, and severe. Mild symptoms include headache, nausea, vomiting, dizziness, and blurred vision; moderate symptoms include syncope, dyspnoea, tachycardia, tachypnea, and rhabdomyolysis; and severe symptoms include palpitations, dysrhythmias, respiratory arrest, cardiac arrest, and coma [6].

Oxygen therapy is the first-line treatment for suspected or confirmed carbon monoxide toxicity, and it is administered through a face mask or, if necessary, an endotracheal tube. The half-life of COHb can be reduced to 40–45 minutes when using 100% FiO_2 through continuous positive airway pressure, and it can be reduced to 20 minutes when using 100% high-flow oxygen therapy [5].

3.2 Hydrogen cyanide toxicity

Hydrogen cyanide, like CO, is a by-product of incomplete combustion, but it is derived from synthetic materials. Similar to CO, hydrogen cyanide enters the cell quickly and inhibits oxidative phosphorylation while promoting anaerobic metabolism [4], inducing a state of 'chemical shock' as it causes tissue hypoxia.

4. Inhalation injury

One of the most difficult tasks in the management of burn patients is determining whether the patient is at risk of inhalation injury because this will play a significant role in the patient's outcome, as this is one of the most important risk factors for the development of ARDS and higher mortality.

4.1 Pathophysiology

Major burns, without a doubt, cause a severe inflammatory response due to tissue destruction and fluid dysregulation. Following a severe burn, an acute phase inflammatory response triggers the release of cytokines and chemokines, which corresponds with a hypermetabolic state, consuming proteins, glucose, and fluid requirement [7]. This translates into initial fluid management in the severely burned patient and a distributive shock, which must be managed with a goal in mind.

The human airway is a highly perfused organ. When there is II, it increases 10–15 times as the hypermetabolic response kicks in, followed by edema of the upper and lower airways (depending on the site of injury), increasing resistance, limiting airflow, and forming a fibrin clot and cast [7]. We may experience significant airway obstruction when this happens, resulting in a ventilation-perfusion mismatch, atelectasis, and hypoxia.

As part of the inflammatory response, edema starts to occur in the upper and lower airways within hours of the burn injury. Then, in the hypermetabolic state, the cardiac output further promotes the airway inflammatory response, causing not only airway edema but also increasing the metabolic demand for analgesic and anesthetic drugs, as well as fluid requirements during the resuscitation phase [7].

This airway compromise, combined with the severe inflammatory response and the need for advanced airway management, makes the respiratory system vulnerable to infections, most notably pneumonia.

Edema, debris, and epithelial destruction eventually form airway casts, causing airway obstruction, high resistance, ventilation-perfusion mismatch, and atelectasis and preventing oxygen and tidal volume from reaching the alveoli, making lung unit recruitment difficult and predisposing the patient to pneumonia, barotrauma, high auto-positive end-expiratory pressure (PEEP), increased plateau pressure and, eventually, ARDS. We can prevent or at least minimize these complications and improve the outcome if we can remove these casts as part of the treatment of inhalation injury [7].

Inhalation injury causes bronchospasm through poorly understood mechanisms, although neuropeptides produced in the submucosa due to inflammation are responsive to aerosolized albuterol or epinephrine, suggesting the origin from a smooth muscle spasm [7].

There is a high airway resistance in the setting for mechanical ventilator management, resulting in auto-PEEP, making maintaining a safe peak pressure and an adequate plateau pressure difficult (**Figure 2**), implying the need for constant recruitment of lung units based on advanced modes of ventilation, as explained later in this chapter.

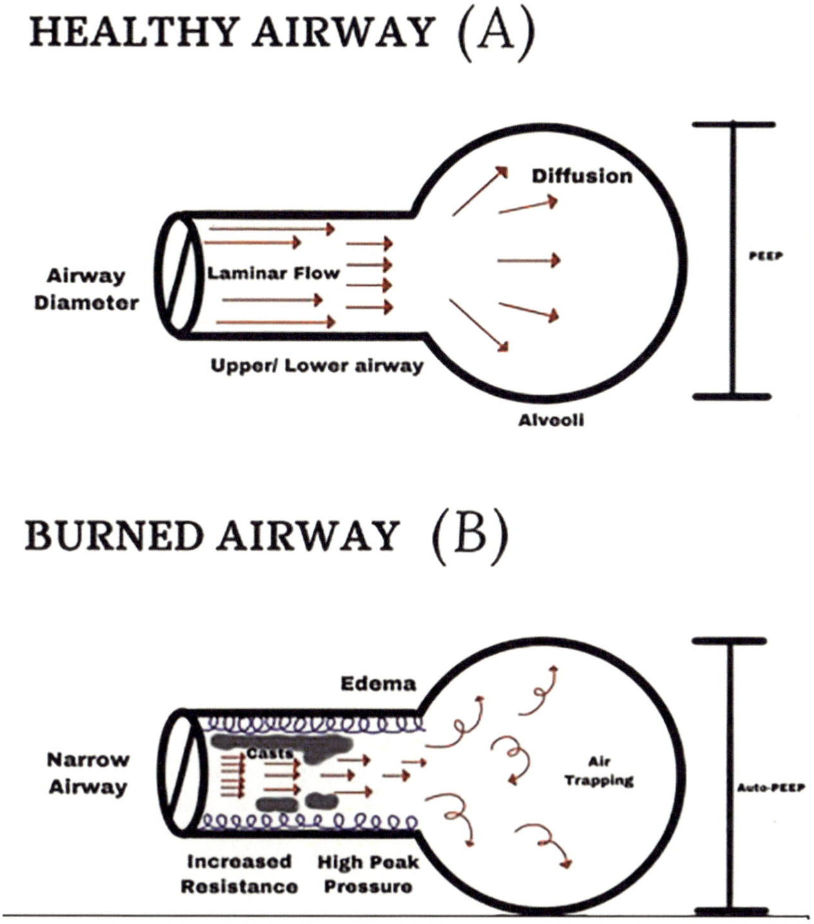

Figure 2.
Changes in the airway of a severely burned patient with inhalation injury.

4.2 Treatment

The most critical measure is determining whether advanced airway management, cervical spine stabilization, and, if necessary, life support is required in a deteriorating airway.

After assessing for a secure airway and preventing CO toxicity from progressing, one can focus on improving dynamics in inhalation injury. Beta 2 agonists aerosolized bronchodilators relax the smooth muscle in the upper and lower airways, reducing airway resistance and allowing a more laminar flow in and out during every ventilation cycle [7].

N-acetylcysteine is a mucolytic agent that aids in the prevention of airway mucus secretion accumulation. However, it is pungent to the airway and may cause bronchospasm, so it should not be used without a bronchodilator [7].

As debris is caused by fibrin cloths, casts, and damaged cells, aerosolized anticoagulants such as heparin have been described to improve lung dynamics [7].

As the purpose of this chapter, we will go over ventilator strategies to improve mortality in severely burned patients, as well as the considerations we must make when managing a severely burned patient under mechanical ventilation.

4.2.1 Fluid management

The fluid management in the severe burn has been of great concern, mostly because of its nature as part of the burn pathophysiology. Burn Shock has been described as an endpoint to dehydration, structure modification of plasma proteins, vascular leak, causing cellular ischemia, and switching to anaerobic metabolism (shock).

Traditionally, classic Parkland Formula has been used to guide fluid management in the burn patient with a TBSA >20%. Nevertheless, recent studies show it is not always precise in improving resuscitation in this specific population. The modern approach to fluid management in the severely burn patient, is aiming for a goal – directed fluid balance, with a tendency to zero fluid accumulation and adequate fluid resuscitation, maintaining urine output between 0.5 and 1.0 mL/kg/hr., thus avoiding over-resuscitation and all the consequences of detrimental mortality such as abdominal compartment syndrome, pulmonary edema, pleural effusion, myocardial edema, poor wound healing, tissue edema, and all these factors lead to sepsis, ultimately ARDS [8, 9].

4.3 Diagnosis

Bronchoscopy has recently been proposed as the gold standard for inhalation injury due to direct observation of the injured tissue. However, there were limitations to this method, such as cost, a lack of equipment in some centers, and a lack of operator expertise. There is also a limitation for reaching distal airways, which may explain the lack of relationship between higher grades of II and higher mortality reported in some studies [10], making it necessary to complete the assessment with imaging testing, such as computed tomography showing parenchymal changes in the lung compatible with II [11]. Due to its limitations, it is not recommended to use it as a single test to diagnose II.

To summarize, the most appropriate approach for effectively diagnosing inhalation injury would be a comprehensive assessment that includes clinical features, demographics, mechanism of burn injury, imaging, and bronchoscopy.

5. Risk for ARDS

There is a controversial relationship between II and ARDS. Some studies claim there is no correlation, whereas others claim it is strongly related. Both II and pneumonia have been shown to increase the risk of moderate and severe ARDS [3]. The Berlin Criteria is an effective tool for determining the severity of burn-related ARDS with or without inhalation injury [3].

Other studies have found that, among other variables and demographics, II is a major factor in the development of ARDS. Thus, the Abbreviated Burn Severity Index (ABSI), a scoring system designed for patients suffering from starch-based powder burns, was developed with a reliable OR and a very high sensitivity and specificity ranging above 9 points in the scoring system [1].

6. Mechanical ventilation management

Multiple studies show that II is a significant risk factor for a prolonged ICU stay, the need for mechanical ventilation, the development of ARDS, pneumonia, and an increase in mortality [10].

6.1 Lung-protective ventilation

Prior to the development of lung-protective ventilation, the mortality rate in patients requiring mechanical ventilation was increasing. Much has been written about improving the outcome of mechanically ventilated patients and reducing the risk of ARDS and ventilator-induced lung injury (VILI). The modern view of ventilator management emphasizes different goals than those described before the 2000s.

The ARDSnet protocol, which specified low-tidal ventilation and a plateau pressure goal, was a significant breakthrough in mechanical ventilation. Each step in lung-protective ventilation is described in detail here.

6.1.1 Tidal volume

The modern recommendation for preventing VILI when it comes to tidal volume (Vt) in ARDS patients is that it be limited to 4–8 ml/kg PBW [12], which has been shown to improve mortality by 22% and increase ventilator-free days as stated in the ARDSnet trial and confirmed by numerous authors. Also, keep the ventilation goals for Vt in mind at all times.

Modern therapeutic tidal volume goals explain the relationship between excessive strain, higher tidal volume, and volutrauma [13].

When there is a tendency for airway collapse and increased resistance, higher tidal volumes pose a risk for air trapping, auto-PEEP, barotrauma, and volutrauma; lower volumes are preferred in inhalation injury.

6.1.2 Positive end expiratory pressure

Prior to the implementation of lung-protective ventilation, higher PEEP was thought to be detrimental to lung homeostasis. Higher PEEP is now known to be essential for preventing atelectasis not only in patients with ARDS but also in healthy surgical patients [14]. According to numerous guidelines and studies, higher PEEP (>5 cmH_2O) improves mortality in patients with moderate to severe ARDS, as well as the length of stay in the ICU [15].

Physiologically, PEEP reduces stress by acting as a buffer to the constant opening and closing of the alveoli, eliminating the need to reach the opening threshold in each respiratory cycle [16]. Of course, there are exceptions to the rule, such as in patients with a fibrotic lung pattern, in which the non-recruitable areas predominate, as higher PEEP is associated with higher mortality [16].

However, higher PEEP (>5 cmH_2O) is an important part of lung-protective ventilation because it has been shown to improve oxygenation and alveolar recruitment, improve mortality and reduce stress to the alveolar unit [12, 13].

Airway resistance and a proclivity for airway collapse in severely burned patients increase the risk of air trapping and, as a result, auto-PEEP and increased effort to ventilate distal lung units. Therefore we can use higher PEEP in severe ARDS for severely burned patients with inhalation injury, so we can avoid or at least minimize air trapping while using lower tidal volumes and respiratory rates.

6.1.3 Plateau pressure

Peak pressure (Ppeak) and plateau pressure (Pplat) differ significantly. Peak pressure is the representation of the pressure in the airway as a unit, without differentiating between small alveolar units and larger airway components. Pplat, in contrast, is the pressure where gas exchange occurs in the lung and the alveoli. Therein lies the importance of maintaining an optimal Pplat while ventilating our patients.

Several studies have set the higher point of Pplat in 30 cmH_2O, or close to 28 cmH_2O, as high Pplat represents increased strain and mortality [12].

As previously stated, the severely burned patient tends to generate high pressure in the lung due to increased resistance in the airway, decreasing compliance. The Pplat must be given special attention to prevent barotrauma in the stiff chest wall and narrow airways of the ventilated, severely burned patients.

6.1.4 Driving pressure

The formula for driving pressure (DP) is plateau pressure minus PEEP, which represents the difference in alveolar pressure at the end of the inspiration (Pplat) and pressure at the end of expiration (PEEP) or, in other words, the changes in alveolar pressure between each cycle of ventilation.

A DP of <15 cmH_2O is expected to minimize lung stress and prevent VILI [12].

DP is one of the best modern predictors of VILI in any type of patient under mechanical ventilation. This influence is explained either by elastance or tidal volume (stress and strain). However, we should always keep its components (Pplat and PEEP) in mind when guiding lung-protective ventilation. As such, the DP could be in a safe range but not them [13].

The burn patient's low lung compliance and stiff chest wall made achieving lower DP values in lung-protective ventilation the most difficult. Most severely burned patients will need to be intubated immediately after the injury and before a chest escharotomy can be performed, so we may have to adjust our parameters as low as possible to truly minimize lung damage and avoid VILI.

6.1.5 FiO_2

FiO_2 should be titrated in any ventilated patient to achieve oxygen and CO_2 goals, but in the case of a burn patient, we must consider the risk of carbon dioxide poisoning, which is a very common acute complication.

Diagnosis and management of carbon dioxide are very important, as they could pose very serious complications. With carboxyhemoglobin half-life and our patients' clinical evidence in mind, we can choose between hyperbaric oxygen therapy (HBOT) and 100% O_2 [6].

Once the carboxyhemoglobin levels have been determined to be safe, we can begin titrating FiO_2 for therapeutic targets such as arterial PO_2 55–88 mmHg, $SatO_2$ 88–95%, and a PCO_2 of ≤50 mmHg for a pH between 7.30 and 7.40 [17].

6.1.6 Mechanical power

Mechanical power is a novel concept that aims to bring together all of the factors that contribute to VILI [18]. Its components are respiratory system elastance, a dynamic measure that represents variations in airway pressure as volume changes in the lung with each cycle; airway resistance, which, as mentioned earlier, is high in the burned airway; and PEEP.

Parameter	Therapeutic Goal
Tidal Volume	4–8 mL/kg of PBW
PEEP	>5 cmH_2O, preferably >10 cmH_2O in ARDS
Pplat	≤28 cmH_2O
Driving Pressure	≤ 15 cmH_2O
Mechanical Power	< 17 J
FiO_2	100% while assessing for CO Poisoning, then titrate to achieve the goal of pO_2
pH	7.30–7.40
pO_2	55–88 mmHg
PCO_2	< 50 mmHg
$SatO_2$	88–95%

Table 1.
Goals for the lung protective ventilation in the severely burned.

Mechanical power represents the energy applied to the lung on a molecular level, and forcing the lung to receive high energy and stress, damaging elastin to a molecular level, increases the risk for ventilator-induced complications [16].

Lowering the mechanical power may be essential to the new lung-protective ventilation strategies, especially in the high resistance, stiff, burned lung developing ARDS, where compliance is unstable and minor changes in the volume represent deteriorating lung pressure.

All these recommendations are summarized in **Table 1**.

6.2 Other alternatives in the ventilator management

6.2.1 High-frequency percussive ventilation (HFPV)

High-frequency percussive ventilation is a pneumatically driven, pressure-limited, time-cycled mode of ventilation. It is an advanced ventilation mode with a promising future in managing ARDS, specifically in the management of burn patients.

A series of studies have shown that it reduces the incidence of ventilator-associated pneumonia (VAP), improves gas exchange, and reduces the need for higher peak pressures with lower tidal volumes [19].

HFPV has not been shown to reduce mortality when compared to low-tidal volume. Still, it improves oxygenation and the number of available alveolar units, so it is now used regularly in burn centers in the United States [20].

6.3 Airway pressure release ventilation (APRV)

Stock et al. first described APRV as a mode for continuous positive airway pressure with deliberate release periods, in which it generates a high pressure (P high) for a long period of time (T high), simulating long alveolar recruitment, followed by a release phase in a lower pressure (P low) during the set release period (T low) (**Figure 3**) [21].

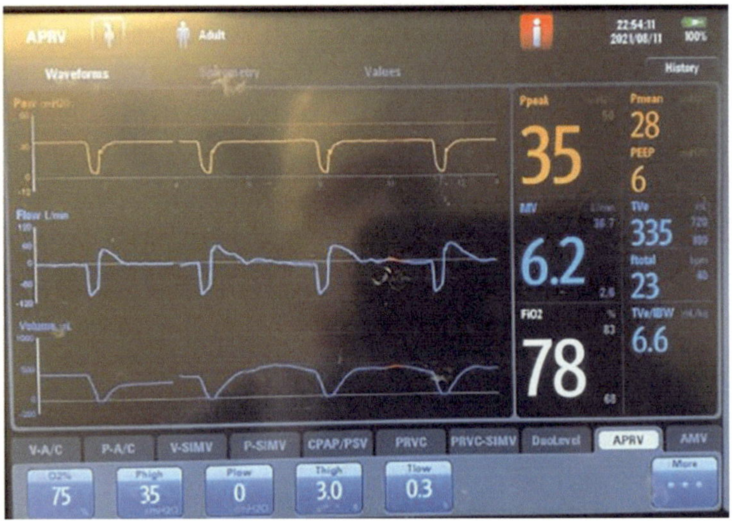

Figure 3.
Mechanically ventilated patient with APRV – TCAV. T high is lower than usual and a T – PEFR of 75%, used as a rescue strategy for a recruitable lung. Courtesy from Pedro González – Noris, MD.

One of the most convenient advantages is the amount of sedation required to maintain this mode. Although in some patients with ARDS, we require a RASS of −3 or −4, this mode requires a RASS of −2, and it is also compatible with prone positioning, which preserves reflexes, favors spontaneous breathing, and reduces the risk for VAP [20, 22]. We could theoretically use this mode in patients with low compliance and poor oxygenation, such as severely burned patients [23].

However, there are some concerns about using this mode, specifically in burn patients. According to some animal studies, the APRV-treated population developed ARDS faster than the conventional ventilation population [20]. In contrast, a retrospective study performed by Foster et al. on burn patients suggests that APRV is a safe ventilation model for these patients [24].

When managing this mode, we must be mindful of some precautions, such as patients with underlying comorbidities who do not tolerate low sedation, commonly neurologically critical patients [21], as well as patients generating auto-PEEP and air trapping [20].

Complementing APRV, time-controlled adaptive ventilation is a method developed to minimize the dynamic alveolar strain by adjusting the delivered breath, focusing on the release phase for the expiratory flow to terminate (EFT) at 75% of the expiratory flow peak (EFP).

The formula $E_{FP} \times 75\% = E_{FT}$ was empirically identified at the bedside as effective at lung stabilization and maintaining open and stable alveoli, resulting in homogeneously ventilated alveoli. This novel ventilation method changes the current approach to mechanical ventilation from arbitrary to personalized and adaptive, but more randomized controlled trials are required [25].

7. Conclusions

The multifactorial causes of ARDS in burn patients are significant. A severely burned patient has an increased inflammatory response after a prolonged hypermetabolic phase that can last longer than usual severe trauma; early management is critical and can dramatically change the outcome.

We must consider ARDS in severely burned patients as a rapidly progressing fibrosis in which we are racing against metabolic, chemical, and physical damage to the respiratory system. If lung-protective ventilation is not achieved in a modern setting, mortality will keep increasing hour by hour.

When it comes to selecting a mode of ventilation for a burn patient, nothing is entirely clear. The outcomes are very similar as long as we achieve the lung-protective ventilation goals. Thus, there is no one-size-fits-all ventilation technique in these situations. We must choose what our patient responds better to and always be aware of complications, how to prevent them and how to solve them.

Acknowledgements

This chapter is made possible in part by the Anesthesiology and the Plastic Surgery team from the Burn Unit of the Traumatology Hospital of Dr. Victorio de la Fuente Narváez in Mexico City for their training on the management of burn patients in critical scenarios.

Thank you to all of the Anesthesia Attending staff and chief of Anesthesia in the Dr. Darío Fernández General Hospital for pushing me to learn more about mechanical ventilation.

Conflict of interest

The authors declare no conflict of interest.

Notes

The figures and tables used in this chapter were photos and diagrams developed by the author and colleagues.

Author details

José Manuel Araiza-Sanchez[1*], Pedro Yasfir González-Noris[2,3],
Juan José Espinoza-Espinosa[4] and Marcos Alfonso Rosas[1]

1 Anesthesiology Resident, Dr. Darío Fernández Fierro General Hospital, Mexico City, Mexico

2 Intensive Care Unit, La Paz General Hospital ISSSTE, La Paz, Mexico

3 Intensive Care Unit, Juan María de Salvatierra General Hospital, La Paz, Mexico

4 Anesthesiologist, Dr. Darío Fernández Fierro General Hospital, Mexico City, Mexico

*Address all correspondence to: manuelmangore@gmail.com

References

[1] Kuan-Hsun L, Chin-Ming C, Yu Kai L, Hao-Yu C, Ta-Wei P, Yuan-Ming T, et al. The abbreviated burn severity index as a predictor of acute respiratory distress syndrome in young individuals with severe flammable starch-based powder burn. Burns. 2018;**44**:1573-1578. DOI: 10.1016/j.burns2018.01.006

[2] Bartels P, Thamm O, Elrod J, Fuchs P, Reinshagen K, Registry GB, et al. The ABSI is dead, long live the ABSI - reliable prediction of survival in burns with a modified abbreviated burn severity index. Burns. 2020;**46**(6):5-7. DOI: 10.1016/j.burns.2020.05.003

[3] Belenkiy S, Buel A, Cannon J, Sine C, Aden J, Henderson J, et al. Acute respiratory distress syndrome in wartime military burns: Application of the Berlin criteria. The Journal of Trauma and Acute Care Surgery. 2013;**76**(3):822-826. DOI: 10.1097/TA.0b013e3182aa2d21

[4] American College of Surgeons. Advanced Trauma Life Support. 2018

[5] Mace S. Challenges and advances in intubation: Rapid sequence intubation. Emergency Medicine Clinics of North America. 2008;**26**:1043-1068

[6] Nañagas K, Penfond S, Kao L. Carbon monoxide toxicity. Emergency Medicine Clinics. 2022;**40**:283-312. DOI: 10.1016/j.emc.2022.01.005

[7] Enkhbaatar P, Pruitt B, Suman O, Mlcak R, Wolf S, Sakurai H, et al. Pathophysiology, research challenges, and clinical management of smoke inhalation injury. The Lancet. 2016;**388**:1437-1446. DOI: 10.1016/S0140-6736(16)31458-1

[8] Dries D, Marini J. Management of critical burn injuries: Recent developments. Korean Journal of Critical Care Medicine. 2017;**32**(1):9-12. DOI: 10.4266/kjccm.2016.00969

[9] Malbrain M et al. Principles of fluid management and stewardship in septic shock: It is time to consider the four D's and the four phases of fluid therapy. Annals of Intensive Care. 2018;**8**:66. DOI: 10.1186/s13613-018-0402-x

[10] Suresh M, Pruskowski K, Rizzo J, Gurney J, Cancio L. Characteristics and outcomes of patients with inhalation injury treated at a military burn center during U.S. combat operations. Burns. 2020;**46**:454-458. DOI: 10.1016/j.burns.2019.08.008

[11] Charles W, Collins D, Mandalia S, Matwala K, Dutt A, Tatlock J, et al. Impact of inhalation injury on outcomes in critically ill burns patients: 12-year experience at a regional burns centre. Burns [Internet]. 2022;**48**:1386-1395. DOI: 10.1016/j.burns.2021.11.018

[12] Fan E. An Official American Thoracic Society/European society of intensive care medicine/Society of critical care medicine clinical practice guideline: Mechanical ventilation in adult patients with acute respiratory distress syndrome. American Journal of Respiratory. 2017;**195**:1253-1263. DOI: 10.1164/rccm.201703-0548ST

[13] Tonetti T, Vasques F, Rapetti F, Maiolo G, Collino F, Romitti F, et al. Driving pressure and mechanical power: New targets for VILI prevention. Annals of Translational Medicine. 2017;**5**(14). DOI: 10.21037/atm.2017.07.08

[14] Young C. Lung-protective ventilation for the surgical patient: International expert panel-based consensus

recommendations. British Journal of Anaesthesia. 2019;**123**:898-913. DOI: 10.1016/j.bja.2019.08.017

[15] Clesson J, Freundlich M, Gunnarsson I, Laake J, Vandvik P, Varpula T, et al. Scandinavian clinical practice guideline on mechanical ventilation in adults with the acute respiratory distress syndrome. Acta Anaesthesiologica Scandinavica. 2014;**59**:286-297. DOI: 10.1111/aas.12449

[16] Marchioni A, Tonelli R, Rossi G, Spagnolo P, Luppi F, Cerri S, et al. Ventilatory support and mechanical properties of the fibrotic lung acting as a "squishy ball". Annals of Intensive Care [Internet]. 2020;**10**(13):2-10. DOI: 10.1186/s13613-020-0632-6

[17] Rademacher P, Maggiore S, Mercat A. Gas exchange in acute respiratory distress syndrome. American Journal of Respiratory care. 2017;**196**(8):964-984. DOI: 10.1164/rccm.201610-2156SO

[18] Gattninoni L et al. Ventilator – Related causes of lung injury: The mechanical power. Intensive Care Medicine. 2016;**42**:1567-1575. DOI: 10.1007/s00134-016-4505-2

[19] Chung K, Cancio L, Wolf S. High-frequency percussive ventilation and low tidal volume ventilation in burns: A randomized controlled trial. Critical Care Medicine. 2010;**38**(10):1970-1976

[20] Folwell JS, Basel AP, Britton GW, Mitchell TA, Rowland MR, Cindass R, et al. Mechanical ventilation strategies in the critically ill burn patient: A practical review for clinicians. European Burn Journal. 2021;**2**:140-151

[21] Ehab D. Airway pressure release ventilation. Annals of Thoracic Medicine. 2007;**2**(4):176-179

[22] Peck M, Koppelman T. Low-tidal-volume ventilation as a strategy to reduce ventilator-associated injury in ALI and ARDS. Journal of Burn Care. 2009;**30**(1):172-173. DOI: 10.1097/BCR.0b013e3181923c32

[23] Mlcak R. Airway pressure release ventilation. Journal of Burn Care. 2009;**30**(1):176-177. DOI: 10.1097/BCR.0b013e3181923c58

[24] Foster K. Use of airway pressure relief ventilation (APRV) in burn patients with and without inhalation injury. Journal of Burn Care. 2021;**42**:S15-S16. DOI: 10.1093/jbcr/irab032.019

[25] Nieman GF, Gatto LA, Andrews P, et al. Prevention and treatment of acute lung injury with time-controlled adaptive ventilation: Physiologically informed modification of airway pressure release ventilation. Annals of Intensive Care. 2020;**10**:3

Section 5

Role of VV-ECMO in Respiratory Failure

Chapter 7

VV-ECMO in Respiratory Insufficiency

Muhammad K. Hayat Syed, Shehabaldin Alqalyoobi, Hillary Vaughan and Salim Surani

Abstract

Extracorporeal membrane oxygenation (ECMO) has advanced significantly in the last few decades. Although not FDA-approved in the United States for respiratory insufficiency, it is widely used to support cardiac and pulmonary function via Venoarterial (VA) and Venovenous (VV) ECMO, respectively. In the patient with worsening respiratory failure VV-ECMO is considered a salvaging therapy that gives patients' lungs time to heal or as a bridge to lung transplant. Clinicians use tools like the Murray score to initiate a referral for VV-ECMO using indices like oxygen requirement, pulmonary compliance, and bilateral opacities. Early referral for VV-ECMO within 7 days of intubation has shown better results. Important factors that are considered in ECMO candidacy are patients' age, comorbid conditions, and chronic conditions that would affect patients' overall longevity. Extracorporeal life support organization (ELSO) gets data from ECMO centers worldwide and has general recommendations for centers guiding treatment and management. During the COVID pandemic, there was a huge surge in acute respiratory distress syndrome (ARDS) and rampant use of VV-ECMO for COVID-ARDS. Data from various centers have helped us understand the appropriate use of VV-ECMO for ARDS and other causes of hypoxic and hypercapnic respiratory failure. Early referral and careful screening for the patient for ECMO are of paramount importance for a better outcome.

Keywords: VV ECMO, ARDS, interstitial lung disease, IPF, AE IPF, ELSO, ECMO

1. Introduction

Extracorporeal membrane oxygenation (ECMO) has allowed treatment for severe cardiac and pulmonary failure using the concept of a heart-lung bypass pump used in cardiothoracic surgeries. ECMO provides mechanical cardiopulmonary support using a circuit consisting of a pump and membrane oxygenator as key components. Venovenous ECMO, known as VV-ECMO, supports patients with severe respiratory failure. It requires the insertion of cannulae and circulating blood through an extracorporeal circuit where it is oxygenated and then returned to the patient. In VV-ECMO, it will be drained from and returned to the venous side of the systemic circulation. In this chapter, we will cover the basic VV-ECMO circulations and cardiac and respiratory physiology. **Figure 1** is showing VV-ECMO Circuit.

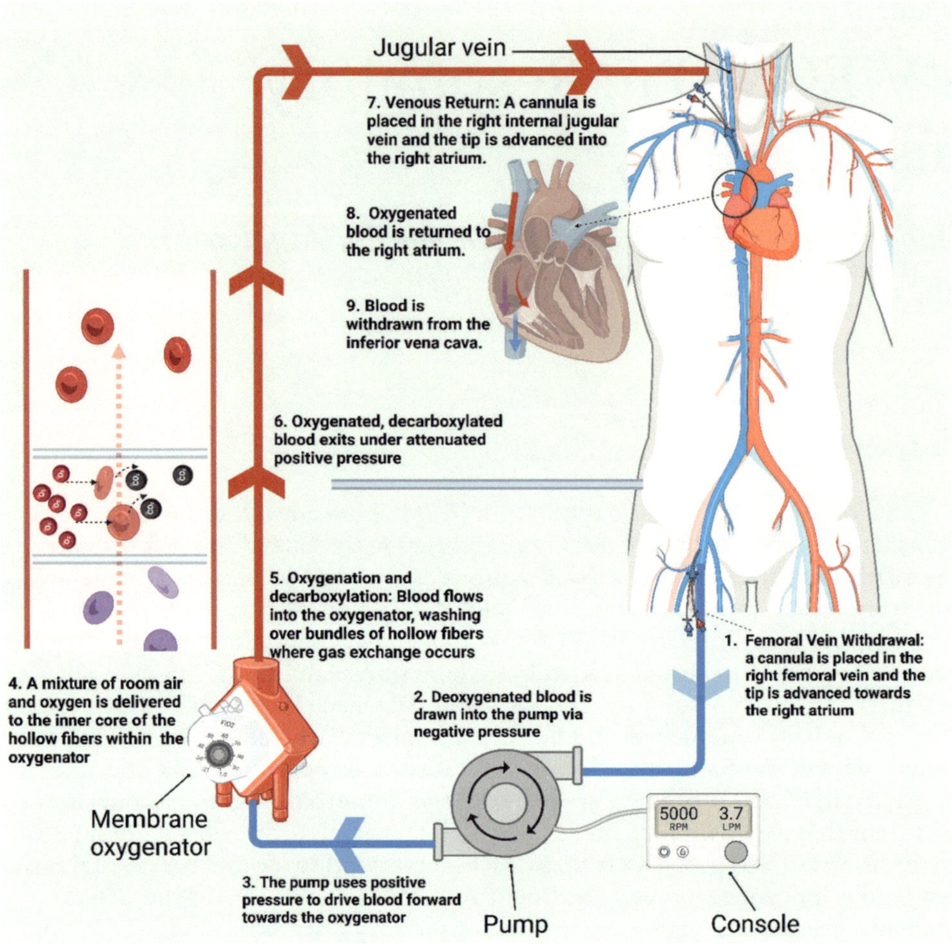

Figure 1.
VV ECMO circuit showing drainage of blood and return to body on venous side after passing through the membrane oxygenator and the pump.

1.1 Oxygen content

Alveolar oxygen partial pressure (PAO_2) is slightly lower than the atmospheric air O_2 ~ 100 mmHg due to the humidification and water content. The arterial oxygen partial pressure (PaO_2) is ~90 mmHg. On the VV-ECMO machine, the venous blood will pass through the gas chamber of the oxygenator (PO_2 ~ 550–600 mmHg, PCO_2 = 0). The oxygen will diffuse from the gas chamber to the blood, while CO_2 will diffuse out. The CO_2 will leave the oxygenator from the outlet. PaO_2 and PCO_2 pre and post-membranes can be analyzed by collecting blood gasses pre and post-membranes [1].

The amount of oxygen in the blood is determined by two main factors: oxygen bound to hemoglobin (98.5%) and dissolved in plasma (1.5%). The total oxygen content of blood is calculated using this equation [2] (CaO_2 arterial oxygen content) as shown in **Table 1**.

CaO_2 = Hb (gm/dl) × 1.34 ml O_2/gm Hb × SaO_2 + (PaO_2 × 0.003 ml O_2/mm Hg/dl) CaO_2 = 15 x 1.34x 1.00 + (90 x 0.003) = 20.37 g/dl
CaO_2 ~ 20 g/dL for a human with normal hemoglobin (15 g/dL), PaO_2 of 90 mmHg, and saturation of 100%. The solubility coefficient of oxygen in plasma is 0.003.
CvO_2 = 15 × 1.34 × 0.75 + (40 × 0.003) = 15.195 g/dl
The CvO2 ~ 15 g/dL for a human with normal hemoglobin (15 g/dL), PvO2 of 40 mmHg, and a saturation of 75%.
DO_2 = CO × CaO_2 DO_2 = HR × SV × CaO_2
The oxygen delivery (DO_2, mL/kg/min) is the amount of oxygen delivered to the tissue (in mL/kg) per unit of time (in min). Normal oxygen delivery equals ~15–25 mL/kg/min (at a normal cardiac output of 5 LPM and arterial oxygen content of 20 g/dL.
O_2 ER = DO_2:VO_2
OThe oxygen extraction ratio of VV-ECMO under normal physiologic conditions is 20–25%.

O_2 ER: Oxygen Extraction Ratio; DO_2: Oxygen Delivery; VO_2: Oxygen consumption, CO: Cardiac output; SV: Stroke volume; HR: Heart Rate.

Table 1.
Arterial and venous oxygen content (CaO_2, CvO_2) and oxygen delivery (DO_2).

These equations apply to the oxygenator on VV-ECMO to calculate the pre-membrane and post-membrane oxygen content. Using the same principle, we can calculate the CvO_2. **Table 1** DO_2 is determined by the oxygen content and the cardiac output (CO) [3] as shown below:

On the other side, oxygen consumption (VO_2, mL/min) is the difference between the arterial and venous oxygen content multiplied by the cardiac output.

1.2 Equation (naive circulation) (oxygen consumption)

The oxygen consumption is approximately 3–5 mL/kg/min. The ratio of DO_2: VO_2 [1] is the oxygen extraction ratio (O_2 ER). Under normal physiologic conditions, O_2 ER is 20–25%. The DO_2 during the ECMO circuit is the product of the oxygen content of the post-oxygenator blood multiplied by the circuit blood flow.

1.3 Equation ECLS (oxygen delivery)

The total DO_2 equals the DO_2 of the naive circulation plus the DO_2 of the ECLS machine. The two circulations are connected in series. In VV-ECMO, usually, the cardiac output of the patient is higher than the ECMO circuit.

$$\text{Equation Total } DO_2 = \text{ECLS } DO_2 + \text{Naive circulation } DO_2 \tag{1}$$

To determine the contribution of the VV-ECMO circulation to the oxygenation of the naive circulation, we divide the blood flow of the circuit by the naive circulation circuit. For example, if the ECMO circuit flow is 3 LPM and the patient's cardiac output is 5 LPM, then 60% of the patient's blood is being oxygenated by the ECMO circuit, and the patient's diseased lung oxygenates 40%.

The carbon dioxide (CO_2) clearance in the ECLS circuit is determined by the sweep gas flow rate (typically between 1 and 11 L). Due to the high solubility of CO_2, it transfers 6 times faster across the membrane faster than oxygen.

2. Indications and contraindications for VV ECMO

The major indication for VV ECMO a severe but potentially reversible respiratory failure without significant heart failure like ARDS. The decision to initiate an ECMO circuit is refractory hypoxemia and/or hypercapnia after maximizing the standard of care. The term "maximizing" care includes prone positioning, the use of neuromuscular agents, and high positive end-expiratory pressure (PEEP) strategy. It might be appropriate to consider inhaled pulmonary vasodilators and recruitment maneuvers. The concept is to provide adequate oxygenation and ventilation in a patient with severe ARDS and, at the same time, rest the lung to promote healing and prevent mechanical Ventilation-Induced lung injury (VILI).

After considering the above measures, if the PaO_2:FiO_2 ratio is <80 mmHg for >6 hours, the PaO_2:FiO_2 ratio is <50 mmHg for >3 hours, or PCO_2 is >60 mmHg (and pH < 7.25) and no contraindications, then ECMO should be considered if the underlying disease process if potentially reversible (i.e., pneumonia) or the ECMO done as a bridge to a pre-planned surgery or intervention (i.e., lung transplant) [1, 4].

These are relative to the ECMO center and patient characteristics and specific situations. Generally, patients should have a reversible condition like an infection or ARDS or should have a destination plan for a lung transplant, and ECMO is used as a bridging therapy. The absolute contraindication for VV-ECMO is the presence of irreversible pathology and patients who are not a candidate for a lung transplant. Relative contraindications include multiorgan failure, irreversible neurologic injury, uncontrolled bleeding or thrombocytopenia or other bleeding tendencies, metastatic cancer, prolonged mechanical ventilation, and advanced age (greater than 65–70).

3. VV-ECMO for COVID-19 ARDS

ECMO played a significant role in the COVID-19 Pandemic. Overall, the approach to select patients and manage VV-ECMO for COVID-19-related respiratory failure is the same as other etiologies of ARDS.

The two major differences in COVID-19-related infections are cardiovascular and other systemic involvement and outcomes. Respiratory involvement has been the major indication for VV-ECMO. However, 20% of COVID-19 patients have experienced cardiac involvement, [3] and about 4% required VA-ECMO configuration [5]. Different mechanisms like thrombosis, pulmonary embolism, direct damage to the cardiac myocytes, severe inflammatory response, and cardiac arrhythmias [6] have resulted in cardiac failure during COVID-19 infection. The short-term outcomes in COVID-19-related ARDS requiring ECLS have evolved during different waves [5]. During the first wave (prior to May 2020), the mortality was 36% and then increased to 52% in the second wave (between May 2020 and December 2020) [5, 7]. Changes in the virus virulence, the introduction of immunosuppressive medications, and the presence of additional bacterial pneumonia might explain this increase in mortality [8]. A cohort of 1035 patients with COVID-19 ARDS patients managed with VVECMO showed an estimated cumulative hospital mortality of 37% [5] and some COVID-19 patients with high D-dimer and low static compliance phenotype had mortality as high as 56% [9]. These COVID-19 phenotypes might benefit from VVECMO.

4. Extracorporeal carbon dioxide removal (ECCO$_2$R) for hypercapnic respiratory failure

The technology behind ECCO$_2$R overlaps with the VV-ECMO circuit. The major difference is the absence of an oxygenator integrated into the membrane lung. This can be achieved with a smaller cannula like a 14–18 Fr. The blood flows from the venous patient site to the pump (flow range: 0–8 L/min) and then to the membrane lung. The membrane lung has two chambers (blood on one side and sweep gas on the other side). The chamber is separated by a semipermeable membrane. CO_2 diffusion across the membrane is gradient dependent. CO_2 removal is more efficient than oxygenation, and a 1–3 lit/min flow is enough to fully remove CO_2 produced by patients, but this flow might not be enough for oxygenation.

The baseline arterial CO_2 is a product of tissue production and lung ventilation. The higher the blood flow, the greater the CO_2 removal. Similarly, the higher the sweep flow, the greater the CO_2 removal. Maintaining the CO_2 gradient ensures the CO_2 diffusion from the blood to the gas chamber in the membrane lung [10, 11]. The determinants of CO_2 removal are baseline arterial CO_2 content, sweep gas flow, blood flow, blood pH, membrane area, and time of transit.

ARDS and chronic obstructive lung disease (COPD) are the major potential indications for ECCO$_2$R use. In ARDS, the protective mechanical ventilation strategy (low tidal volume, 6 ml/kg of ideal body weight) reduces the risk of VILI, and Respiratory acidosis is a common side effect of this strategy. ECCO$_2$R can be used to assist in ventilation, allowing ultra-protective ventilation (4 ml/kg of ideal body weight) in ARDS patients [12]. This means the damaging [13] plateau pressure, driving pressure, and mechanical power can be kept in an acceptable range [14].

COPD is another potential indication for ECCO$_2$R use. The standard of care suggests the use of noninvasive mechanical ventilation (NIV) to reduce the rate of invasive mechanical ventilation (IMV). However, up to 25% of patients with COPD exacerbation will fail NIV [15]. In this patient population, ECCO$_2$R is considered an additional intervention to prevent IMV.

5. VV ECMO configuration, cannulation and site selection

5.1 Configuration and cannulation site

For VV ECMO, deoxygenated blood is drained from the venous side of the circulation, and oxygenated blood is returned to the venous side or directly into the right atrium and sometimes in the right ventricle (helpful in right heart failure patients). Dual site cannulation IJ-Fem or Fem-Fem with one catheter in Internal Jugular and the other in the Femoral or both in Femoral Veins, respectively. These are more invasive, limiting patient ambulation. Single site dual lumen catheter is accessed via the right IJ vein and is designed to have drainage ports (proximal and distal) to be positioned in IVC and SVC. A return port is in the middle of the catheter that is directed toward

	Cannulation Configuration	Drainage Site	Return Site
1	Single Site Dual Lumen Catheter	IVC and SVC	Right atrium
2	Dual Site Single Lumen	Internal Jugular Vein/ Subclavian	Femoral Veins
3		Femoral Vein	Femoral Vein

Table 2.
Cannulation configuration types.

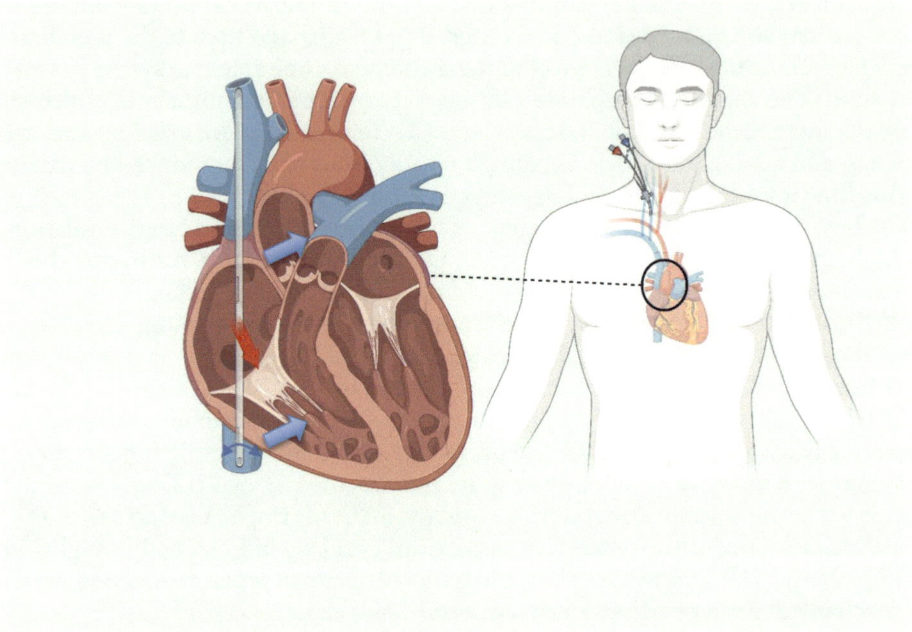

Figure 2.
Single site dual lumen catheter with blue arrows shows drainage of blood to the ECMO circuit and red arrow indicating the return of oxygenated blood into the right atrium.

the tricuspid valve using transesophageal echocardiogram (TEE) and fluoroscopy. Although single-site cannulation is less invasive and allows patient ambulation, the cannula must be sutured and secured carefully, and slight rotation or neck movement can dislodge the ports causing issues. The details of the cannulation configuration types, drainage and return sites are shown in **Table 2**.

5.2 VV ECMO vs. VA ECMO

Single Site Cannulation using Bicaval dual lumen cannula (Avalon) with blue drainage apertures both in SVC and IVC and red return aperture directed toward the tricuspid valve (**Figure 2**).

Two-site cannulation (IJ-Fem) with drainage via femoral access catheter in IVC and return of oxygenated blood to SVC via internal jugular (IJ)/subclavian access (**Figure 3**) [16].

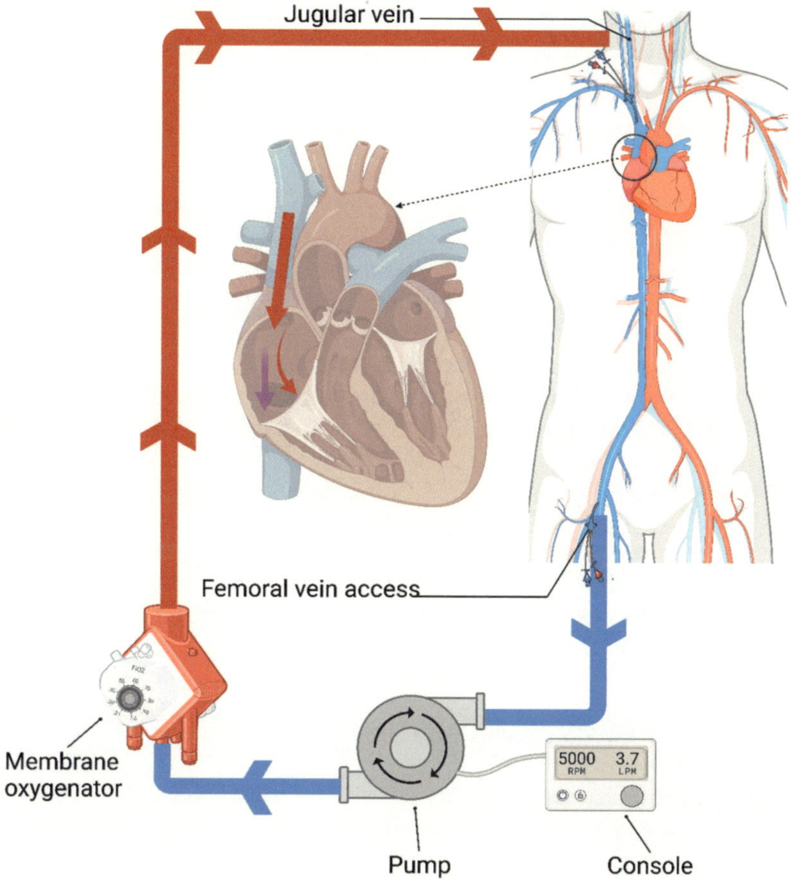

Figure 3.
Dual catheter dual-site configuration.

5.2.1 Difference in indication

VV ECMO is for respiratory failure alone. When we have cardiac failure, we need to use VA ECMO. In VA ECMO, the return cannula is placed in the arterial circulation, i.e., bypassing the heart and lungs. Some commonly used sites are the femoral artery, axillary or subclavian artery. In VV ECMO, the return cannula is placed on the venous side and is pumped by the heart. VV ECMO does not provide any cardiac support directly. However, it may improve hemodynamics by improving hypoxia and acidosis and indirectly improving right and left ventricular function. Placing VA ECMO configuration with normal LVEF will result in complications like north–south syndrome with the heart and ECMO pump forcing blood in opposite directions.

6. Ventilator management on ECMO

While on VV ECMO, the ventilator settings are adjusted to allow lung healing and minimize VILI in the already damaged lung. The goal is to provide oxygenation via the ECMO circuit and not through native lungs. Data from landmark trials [17, 18] have been used to guide ventilator settings. A commonly used setting is pressure support of 10 cmH_2O, PEEP of ≥10 cmH_2O, respiratory rate of 10, and FiO_2 of 0.3 [4]. Other Modes are also used but keeping the tidal volume low so that plateau pressure < 20–25 cm H_2O.

6.1 Extubation while on VV ECMO

In patients who do not have a shock, multiorgan failure and are somewhat stable on supportive care, planned extubation while on VV-ECMO can be considered. Extubation helps decrease sedative medications, improve patients' communication and physical therapy, and decrease ventilator-associated complications. However, patients should be on minimal vent settings (P/F < 0.4 PEEP ~5), able to protect the airway and clear secretions. After extubation, there is a risk of failure and reintubation along with increased work of breathing, so patients should be closely monitored. Post-extubation sweep gas might need to be adjusted depending on arterial blood gas.

6.2 Tracheostomy

Some patients tolerate extubation on ECMO well. Others may develop tachypnea, causing increased work breathing leading to possible reintubation or lung [19]. Tracheostomy can be considered for the patient on prolonged ECMO >10 days and has failed extubation.

7. Complications of VV-ECMO and management

7.1 Vascular complications

7.1.1 Bleeding

By far, bleeding and thrombosis are the most common complication of ECMO. Bleeding is mainly because of the need for anticoagulation to prevent circuit thrombosis. The most common sites are gastrointestinal, cannulae insertion sites, and intracranial bleeds.

Retroperitoneal bleed can happen when the cannula is inserted at the groin site.

7.1.2 Circuit thrombosis

Thrombosis-resistant circuits decrease the chances of circuit thrombosis, but systemic anticoagulation is mandatory.

7.1.3 Systemic thromboembolism

Venous thrombosis and thromboembolism (VTE) are common in patients with VV-ECMO, with incidences reported as low as 10% [20] to as high as 42% [21] even with full anticoagulation. Locations of VTE include upper and lower extremity VTE, cannulation site, and pulmonary emboli. Factors favoring VTE are longer time on ECMO, low pump speed and low blood flow velocity, cannula malposition, kinks, larger bore cannulae, partial thromboplastin time < 50, elevated D dimers, and patients with COVID-19 infections [22].

7.1.4 Cannulation related complications

A systematic review [23] reports a 7% complication rate during cannulation for VV ECMO in 12,800 patients reported in 33 studies. Other less frequently seen complications include catheter site infection, Aneurysms, and pseudoaneurysms [23].

7.2 Oxygenator dysfunction

As the circuit ages, its oxygenator starts to develop microthrombi, leading to a gradual decrease in its efficacy.

7.3 Recirculation and cannula malposition

Recirculation is the phenomenon when oxygenated blood returning to the body is aspirated back by the drainage cannula without passing through systemic circulation, decreasing the efficacy of ECMO. It more commonly happens in single-site ECMO configurations or where the drainage and return cannulae are in proximity. One way of estimating the recirculation fraction is using SvO_2.

$$\text{Recirculation}\,(\%) = (\text{SpreO}_2 - SvO_2)\,/\,(\text{SpostO}_2 - SvO_2) \times 100 \qquad (2)$$

SvO_2 is central venous oxygen saturation in IVC/SVC. When the recirculation is high enough that it requires higher ECMO support, measures are taken to decrease it. Increasing the distance between drainage and return cannulae, adding an additional drainage cannula at a second site, using dual lumen cannula, adjusting the position of cannula/cannulae, and decreasing the pump speed [16] or upsizing the cannulae french can help reduce the recirculation fraction to an acceptable level.

Cannula malposition may occur during patient turns, skincare, or ambulation. This can lead to increased recirculation, patient desaturation, or increased ECMO support. This requires correction using echocardiography transthoracic (TTE), transesophageal (TEE), and/or fluoroscopy to reposition the cannula to the optimum position.

7.4 Neurologic complications

7.4.1 ICH

Intracranial hemorrhages (ICH) are the most common neurologic complication of VV ECMO with high mortality. The most common types of ICH are subarachnoid hemorrhage and intraparenchymal hemorrhage. Most of these are reported to have occurred earlier, within 6–24 hours of ECMO initiation.

7.4.2 Long-term complications

Post-ECMO patients can experience anxiety, depression, and post-traumatic stress. Cognitive deficits and psychiatric symptoms can affect the quality of life. It is important for ECMO survivors to have neuroimaging post-decannulation and follow-up outpatient to screen for possible neuropsychiatric issues.

1.	Sepsis	26.1%
2.	Acute Renal Injury	24.7%
3.	Multiorgan failure	24.7%
4.	Cannulation complications	6.6%
5.	Neurologic complication	6.9%

Table 3.
Incidence of complications in a meta-analysis of 12,800 VV-ECMO patients [23].

In addition to neuroimaging, transcranial dopplers, Pupil index, EEG, and Cerebral infrared spectroscopy can be used to monitor for neurologic complications [24].

Other complications included Infections and Sepsis, likely pneumonia, cannulation site infection, bacteremia, Acute renal failure requiring renal replacement therapy, liver dysfunction, hemolysis, and disseminated intravascular coagulation (DIC). The incidence of complications in a meta-analysis of 12,800 VV-ECMO patients are described in **Table 3** [23].

8. Decannulation/weaning of VV-ECMO

Weaning of VV-ECMO is based on multiple factors like underlying lung pathology, radiographic clearance, lung compliance, other organs' functions, and blood oxygen and carbon dioxide levels. The timing of weaning is a delicate balance between an "optimal" state and "resolution," knowing the risk of ECMO complications.

The basic weaning approach is to gradually reduce the pump flow to a minimum and reassess the patient. One way is to reduce the flow to about 1 L/min in an adult ECMO circuit. Another way is to keep the flow above 3 L/min (to reduce the risk of thrombosis). If the patients remain stable after weaning the sweep gas and FiO_2%, then consideration for a formal weaning trial should be given.

The oxygenation response test is an indicator of lung readiness for weaning of ECMO. This is done by increasing the ventilator FiO_2 to 1.0 and the peripheral saturations to >95%. The sweep gas is weaning as well in response to carbon dioxide levels. It is acceptable to keep the patient in mild respiratory acidosis (pH 7.25–7.35).

After performing the above measure, the formal trial is started by initiating lung protective ventilation. We disconnect the sweep gas from the oxygenator and assess the arterial blood gas every 20–30 mins. The ventilator is adjusted accordingly. The satisfactory arterial blood gas (ABG) means arterial PO_2 > 60 mmHg on lung protective ventilation (TV < 6 ml/kg of IBW, and peak inspiratory pressure < 25 cm/H_2O and FiO_2 < 0.6). If ABG is satisfactory, the blood flow through the circuit is maintained for a period of 2–4 hours to ensure stable organ function. Decannulation is considered if organ function remains stable. If ABG is not satisfactory, then sweep gas should be reconnected, and the patient should be evaluated.

9. Duration of ECMO

Expectations should be set with patients and/or families before initiation of ECMO. This should include a discussion about discontinuing ECMO in case of no recovery in a reasonable time period or if due to any because there is no chance of meaningful survival [25]. Usually, durations last around 2–4 weeks but may vary in centers and regions based on resources and patient characteristics. The pooled average of ~10 days on VV ECMO and about ~25 days of ICU length of stay [23]. Like any other severe critical care illness, patients who were on VVECMO might develop similar deconditioning and psychosocial problems requiring evaluation and therapy.

10. Evidence-based VVECMO outcomes

Many studies are looking at it [26]. A retrospective analysis found better 6-month survival in ECMO-ARDS out of 90 patients. There was great interest in VV ECMO use during the H1N1 pandemic, and then the Cesar trail [17] in the UK, showed a 63% 6-month survival with VV ECMO as compared to 47% with conventional treatment of ARDS. However, 25% of patients referred to the ECMO centers never received treatment. Data from this trial have convinced physicians to make early referrals to ECMO centers in severe ARDS patients. Severe ARDS itself has a mortality of ~45%. A meta-analysis of 33 VV ECMO studies with 12,800 patients showed single-arm meta-analysis mortality of 41% [23]. A subsequent EOLIA trial was stopped for futility. However, a post hoc Bayesian analysis [27] and a meta-analysis [28, 29] of both EOLIA and CESAR trials supported the use of VV ECMO in expert centers for severe ARDS with persistent hypoxemia after being treated with standard therapy for ARDS.

11. Conclusion

VV ECMO is a great tool that can help select patients with severe respiratory failure as they recover and possibly prevent adverse outcomes and as a bridge to transplant therapy for end-stage pulmonary disease patients' pulmonary fibrosis, cystic fibrosis, COPD, etc., after they have failed conventional, evidence-based ARDS therapies like prone ventilation and low tidal volumes. Early referral for VV ECMO to expert centers and careful selection of patients are key to better patient outcomes.

Acknowledgements

Hillary M. Vaughan for creating figures and tables for this chapter.

Conflict of interests

None were reported by the authors.

Author details

Muhammad K. Hayat Syed[1], Shehabaldin Alqalyoobi[2], Hillary Vaughan[1] and Salim Surani[3*]

1 Baylor College of Medicine, Houston, Texas, USA

2 East Carolina University, North Carolina, USA

3 Texas A&M University, College Station, Texas, USA

*Address all correspondence to: srsurani@hotmail.com

References

[1] Tonna JE, Abrams D, Brodie D, Greenwood JC, Rubio Mateo-Sidron JA, Usman A, et al. Management of Adult Patients Supported with Venovenous extracorporeal membrane oxygenation (VV ECMO): Guideline from the extracorporeal life support organization (ELSO). ASAIO Journal. 2021;**67**(6):601-610

[2] Monnet X, Julien F, Ait-Hamou N, Lequoy M, Gosset C, Jozwiak M, et al. Lactate and venoarterial carbon dioxide difference/arterial-venous oxygen difference ratio, but not central venous oxygen saturation, predict increase in oxygen consumption in fluid responders. Critical Care Medicine. 2013;**41**(6):1412-1420

[3] Guzik TJ, Mohiddin SA, Dimarco A, Patel V, Savvatis K, Marelli-Berg FM, et al. COVID-19 and the cardiovascular system: Implications for risk assessment, diagnosis, and treatment options. Cardiovascular Research. 2020;**116**(10):1666-1687

[4] Combes A, Schmidt M, Hodgson CL, Fan E, Ferguson ND, Fraser JF, et al. Extracorporeal life support for adults with acute respiratory distress syndrome. Intensive Care Medicine. 2020;**46**(12):2464-2476

[5] Barbaro RP, MacLaren G, Boonstra PS, Combes A, Agerstrand C, Annich G, et al. Extracorporeal membrane oxygenation for COVID-19: Evolving outcomes from the international extracorporeal life support organization registry. Lancet. 2021;**398**(10307):1230-1238

[6] Shafi AMA, Shaikh SA, Shirke MM, Iddawela S, Harky A. Cardiac manifestations in COVID-19 patients-a systematic review. Journal of Cardiac Surgery. 2020;**35**(8):1988-2008

[7] Schmidt M, Langouet E, Hajage D, James SA, Chommeloux J, Brechot N, et al. Evolving outcomes of extracorporeal membrane oxygenation support for severe COVID-19 ARDS in Sorbonne hospitals, Paris. Critical Care. 2021;**25**(1):355

[8] Dognon N, Gaudet A, Parmentier-Decrucq E, Normandin S, Vincentelli A, Moussa M, et al. Extracorporeal membrane oxygenation for COVID 2019-acute respiratory distress syndrome: Comparison between first and second waves (stage 2). Journal of Clinical Medicine. 2021;**10**(21):4839

[9] Grasselli G, Tonetti T, Protti A, Langer T, Girardis M, Bellani G, et al. Pathophysiology of COVID-19-associated acute respiratory distress syndrome: A multicentre prospective observational study. The Lancet Respiratory Medicine. 2020;**8**(12):1201-1208

[10] Boyle AJ, Sklar MC, McNamee JJ, Brodie D, Slutsky AS, Brochard L, et al. Extracorporeal carbon dioxide removal for lowering the risk of mechanical ventilation: Research questions and clinical potential for the future. The Lancet Respiratory Medicine. 2018;**6**(11):874-884

[11] Schmidt M, Tachon G, Devilliers C, Muller G, Hekimian G, Brechot N, et al. Blood oxygenation and decarboxylation determinants during venovenous ECMO for respiratory failure in adults. Intensive Care Medicine. 2013;**39**(5):838-846

[12] Combes A, Fanelli V, Pham T, Ranieri VM. European Society of Intensive Care Medicine Trials G,

the strategy of ultra-protective lung ventilation with extracorporeal CORfN-OmtsAi. Feasibility and safety of extracorporeal CO(2) removal to enhance protective ventilation in acute respiratory distress syndrome: The SUPERNOVA study. Intensive Care Medicine. 2019;**45**(5):592-600

[13] Rocco PRM, Silva PL, Samary CS, Hayat Syed MK, Marini JJ. Elastic power but not driving power is the key promoter of ventilator-induced lung injury in experimental acute respiratory distress syndrome. Critical Care. 2020;**24**(1):284

[14] Goligher EC, Amato MBP, Slutsky AS. Applying precision medicine to trial design using physiology. Extracorporeal CO(2) removal for acute respiratory distress syndrome. American Journal of Respiratory and Critical Care Medicine. 2017;**196**(5):558-568

[15] Phua J, Kong K, Lee KH, Shen L, Lim TK. Noninvasive ventilation in hypercapnic acute respiratory failure due to chronic obstructive pulmonary disease vs. other conditions: Effectiveness and predictors of failure. Intensive Care Medicine. 2005;**31**(4):533-539

[16] Abrams D, Bacchetta M, Brodie D. Recirculation in venovenous extracorporeal membrane oxygenation. ASAIO Journal. 2015;**61**(2):115-121

[17] Peek GJ, Clemens F, Elbourne D, Firmin R, Hardy P, Hibbert C, et al. CESAR: Conventional ventilatory support vs extracorporeal membrane oxygenation for severe adult respiratory failure. BMC Health Services Research. 2006;**6**:163

[18] Combes A, Hajage D, Capellier G, Demoule A, Lavoué S, Guervilly C, et al. Extracorporeal membrane oxygenation for severe acute respiratory distress syndrome. The New England Journal of Medicine. 2018;**378**(21):1965-1975

[19] Syed MKH, Selickman J, Evans MD, Dries D, Marini JJ. Elastic power of mechanical ventilation in morbid obesity and severe hypoxemia. Respiratory Care. 2020;**66**:626-634

[20] Zangrillo A, Biondi-Zoccai G, Landoni G, Frati G, Patroniti N, Pesenti A, et al. Extracorporeal membrane oxygenation (ECMO) in patients with H1N1 influenza infection: A systematic review and meta-analysis including 8 studies and 266 patients receiving ECMO. Critical Care. 2013;**17**(1):R30

[21] Trudzinski FC, Minko P, Rapp D, Fähndrich S, Haake H, Haab M. et al, Runtime and aPTT predict venous thrombosis and thromboembolism in patients on extracorporeal membrane oxygenation: A retrospective analysis. Annals of Intensive Care. 2016;**6**(1):66

[22] Abruzzo A, Gorantla V, Thomas SE. Venous thromboembolic events in the setting of extracorporeal membrane oxygenation support in adults: A systematic review. Thrombosis Research. 2022;**212**:58-71

[23] Kim JH, Pieri M, Landoni G, Scandroglio AM, Calabrò MG, Fominskiy E, et al. Venovenous ECMO treatment, outcomes, and complications in adults according to large case series: A systematic review. The International Journal of Artificial Organs. 2021;**44**(7):481-488

[24] Zhang H, Xu J, Yang X, Zou X, Shu H, Liu Z, et al. Narrative review of neurologic complications in adults on ECMO: Prevalence, risks, outcomes, and prevention strategies. Frontiers in Medicine. 2021;**8**:713333

[25] Bein T, Brodie D. Understanding ethical decisions for patients on

extracorporeal life support. Intensive Care Medicine. 2017;**43**(10):1510-1511

[26] Tsai H-C, Chang C-H, Tsai F-C, Fan P-C, Juan K-C, Lin C-Y, et al. Acute respiratory distress syndrome with and without extracorporeal membrane oxygenation: A score matched study. The Annals of Thoracic Surgery. 2015;**100**(2):458-464

[27] Goligher EC, Tomlinson G, Hajage D, Wijeysundera DN, Fan E, Jüni P, et al. Extracorporeal membrane oxygenation for severe acute respiratory distress syndrome and posterior probability of mortality benefit in a post hoc Bayesian analysis of a randomized clinical trial. Journal of the American Medical Association. 2018;**320**(21):2251-2259

[28] Munshi L, Walkey A, Goligher E, Pham T, Uleryk EM, Fan E. Venovenous extracorporeal membrane oxygenation for acute respiratory distress syndrome: A systematic review and meta-analysis. The Lancet Respiratory Medicine. 2019;**7**(2):163-172

[29] Combes A, Peek GJ, Hajage D, Hardy P, Abrams D, Schmidt M, et al. ECMO for severe ARDS: Systematic review and individual patient data meta-analysis. Intensive Care Medicine. 2020;**46**(11):2048-2057